Ticket Partner 41

MW00447033

Perfect Partners™

Make Your Hopes & Dreams for

a Great Marriage Come True

Books by Carolyn & Wes Huff

Perfect Partners™
Make Your Hopes & Dreams for a
Great Marriage Come True

Perfect Partners™
Find Your Perfect Partner Step-By-Step

Perfect Partners™
When You Think You've Found Your Perfect
Partner Step-By-Step

Perfect Partners™
Should You Stay or Should You Leave?
Step-By-Step

Perfect Partners™

Make Your Hopes & Dreams for a Great Marriage Come True

Carolyn & Wes Huff

Empowerment Solutions, Inc.,
Severna Park, Maryland 21146

Printed in the United States of America

For information address:

Empowerment Solutions, Inc.
550 M Ritchie Highway
Suite 142
Severna Park, MD 21146

Library of Congress Cataloging-in-Publication Data

Huff, Carolyn & Wes Huff
Perfect Partners™: Make Your Hopes & Dreams for a Great Marriage Come True / Carolyn & Wes Huff

ISBN 1-891336-00-2 $24.95 (Hard Cover)

Library of Congress Catalog Card Number: 97-95016

Cover Designed by Cherry Hepburn, Putnam & Smith, 12309 Moorpark Street, Suite #3, Studio City, CA 91604, (818) 505-1104
Book printed and bound by BookCrafters, Chelsea, MI 48118
Distribution by BookMasters Inc., Mansfield, OH 44905

FIRST EDITION

To God: It has been our mission to bring your love into this world. Thank you for allowing us to succeed in our way.

To Ryan & Amanda: You showed us that great marriages are humanly possible.

To Jeff & Tracey and Todd & Alysa: You wanted a great marriage and got it, too.

To Jennie: We love you and wish you the best.

To David: You're on your way. You can have it all if you want it.

To Wes, From Carolyn: You made it possible for me. Loving you is easy. Loving you is a gift to me.

To Carolyn, From Wes: You are the one I've been looking for all of my life.

To Carolyn's patients: Thank you. Sharing in your lives was a gift to me.

To Stella: Your belief in me came at a turning point in my life. Thank you for being my teacher in the truest sense of the word. I'll never forget what you did for me. Love, Carolyn

To our teachers who missed the mark: Your lives would change for the better if you only realized that you are the student.

To all that thought you were our student, you were really our teacher. And to all that thought you were our teacher, you were really our student.

This book is for you.

Carolyn & Wes

Table of Contents

Acknowledgments

Numerous people helped us birth this book. We'd like to take this opportunity to thank each and every one of them.

When we started this endeavor many people told us we'd never get a publisher without an agent and that no agent would be interested unless we'd already published. Fortunately, we didn't listen to those people. We did search for an agent and of 16 agents we queried eight wanted to see our work. We chose one of them. Ken Atchity agreed to help us sell our book.

Ken and his editors helped us with so many aspects of the book it's difficult to recount. We feel deeply appreciative to Ken, Monica Faulkner, and John Shapiro for all of their help. Thank you very much.

And then Ken introduced us to someone that has helped us in a hundred ways. Devon Blaine, our publicist, of The Blaine Group, and her staff have supported, inspired, and promoted us. We are very grateful.

We have wonderful covers for this book and our workbooks because of Devon and an artist she referred us to. Cherry Hepburn of

Putnam & Smith designed our covers. We thank you for your creative ideas and all of your hard work.

As novice authors and publishers, we had much to learn. Angie Locke and Jean Schroeder of BookCrafters, Inc. have guided us through the maze of pre-press and printing. And Shelley Sapyta of BookMasters, Inc. has arranged for all of our order fulfillment needs. Thank you for your guidance and attention.

A big thank you to two special friends in the publishing business and their daughter, Alysa Dearborn. Alysa is our wonderful daughter-in-law – Carolyn's son's perfect partner. Her parents, Jim and Mary Pruett, are publishers in Boulder, Colorado and have given us help whenever we've asked. When we needed to learn more about the business of publishing, they answered our questions. Mary gave vital information about small publishers to Alysa to forward to us.

All of our children and three of their spouses have given us valuable feedback at different times and we thank them for that.

A variety of friends and family have encouraged us all along the way.

A hearty thanks to you all.

Introduction

Christie started therapy saying, "One minute I feel relieved that he finally wants to get married, the next I can't believe I'm going to marry someone who proposed to me by saying, 'We might as well.' Most of the time I feel disappointed; then I start scolding myself for wanting too much. What's the matter with me? Maybe I'm selfish."

Arnie wanted help handling his obsession with Becky. He said, "Both of us went into this relationship agreeing just to have fun. I was fine with that, but Becky started doing things that led me to believe she wanted more. And I liked that too. She seemed like a dream come true. But as soon as I started getting more serious, she dumped me. I'm completely confused. What'd I do wrong?"

Christie and Arnie were victims of the prevailing myths about dating and marriage: Relationships are never perfect, so do your best to make what you already have work. Christie and Arnie needed to reject the idea that mismatches are natural and to discover the right tools and the right attitudes for finding their perfect partners.

Patent Pending

The process that you are going to read about in this book has, a first time ever, for its kind, patent pending.

A few months ago our patent attorney, Larry Guffey, Baltimore, Maryland, filed a patent application for our method for providing instruction on how an individual can optimally select a perfect marriage partner.

Problems in love and marriage have existed since the beginning of time. Cynical quotes about love and marriage have been recorded dating back to the 1500's. Many believe religious teaching perpetuated about the Garden of Eden tend to show that love and sex cause nothing but trouble. The extent of psychological anguish and pain due to problems in love and marriage appear to be at all-time record levels in American society.

Relatively recent attempts at no fault divorce appear to be having little beneficial effect. Divorce on demand actually appears to be reinforcing the now all-to-common belief that one can never find anyone exactly right, so one must always have an escape hatch in any marriage. The increasing percentage of people living together outside of marriage is further evidence of the widespread nature of this belief.

Today's popular press contains many publications that offer advice on this matter. Most of these tend to be "relationship" oriented methods. Despite all of this relationship oriented information, the need continues to exist for a method that can better help people find their perfect marriage partners. This is evidenced by estimates of over 50 million Americans who currently are unhappily married, apparently not having selected their perfect marriage partners.

Our invention is directed at satisfying the need stated above.

The fact that so many new methods are being created to address the problems of love and marriage suggests a much sought after solution. Furthermore, the magnitude of these problems and the efforts being expended to diminish them imply that the utility of such a solution would be of great practical importance to many facets of American life – having significant sociological and technological impacts resulting from individuals' applying our methods to significantly alter their actions and the physical world around them.

We believe that there are a select number of individual core values and behavior characteristics – the 16 differences that make a difference – in which significant differences between the partners cannot be tolerated if a successful, loving marriage is to ensue. Asking oneself or a potential partner to accept significant differences in these individual core values and behavior characteristics compromises one's integrity. Unfortunately, most people cannot just agree to disagree on these differences, since marriage, with its close proximity, just intensifies these differences that are continually stressed in everyday life. How can you compromise and negotiate your integrity on a daily basis without harm? You shouldn't have to give up yourself to be married. In the event that a couple does agree to disagree, the best marriage for which you can hope is a marriage of convenience. That isn't good enough.

When You Find Your Perfect Partner

When you find your perfect partner – someone who shares your world view, someone who shares your expectations and desires – you'll light up. Your joy will spread to every dimension of your life. You'll discover passion, intimacy, and trust; you'll also find fun and relief from the work of life and, therefore, create the best environment for raising competent, happy children.

Conventional wisdom would have you believe that you'll never find that perfect partner, that no one person can completely satisfy you, and that you'll always have to work hard to make a relationship work. Most books about dating and relationships accept the belief that you'll ultimately have to settle for someone who is less than a perfect match and emphasize the need to improve your relationship skills. But this reliance on conflict resolution has left us with a 50 percent divorce rate.

Our book dramatically breaks with authors who advocate working hard to make a relationship work. We believe that your challenge isn't to understand, accept, and appreciate your differences within marriage; your challenge is to find the perfect partner.

Perfect Partners is a guide for finding your perfect partner for a great marriage.

We've developed a practical approach toward dating and marriage that eliminates the need for guesswork, conflict, and pain by:

-Challenging the myth of marriage as hard work
-Defining bad, mediocre, and great marriages
-Encouraging you to know yourself and what you want
-Identifying 16 differences that make a difference on which you must closely match your mate
-Providing practical techniques for marketing yourself
-Providing five crucial questions to ask yourself before you decide to fall in love
-Presenting a detailed, real-life example of great sex

We know this process from the inside out. As a practicing nurse psychotherapist and a pragmatic businessman who've survived the turmoil of hit-or-miss relationships, we've worked through this process ourselves and have helped hundreds of clients do the same. The results have been strong, healthy marriages and the avoidance of differences that make a real difference.

Perfect Partners speaks from professional and lay, female and male points of view. It offers field-tested advice to:

-Singles looking for meaningful, lifelong

marriages
-Divorcés who want to avoid repeating previous mistakes
-Married couples who wish to assess the potential of their relationships

Readers will find this book exciting and life-transforming because:

-Our comprehensive plan for finding the perfect partner will help them find lifelong happiness in a great marriage
-We show readers that great marriages do exist – that they need not settle for an "okay" relationship they'll have to work at for the rest of their life
-Our personal accounts and other examples will convince readers that "If Wes and Carolyn and others have done it, I can too!"

Although we acknowledge the importance of relationship skills and highly recommend getting really good at resolving conflicts, we feel you can drastically reduce the need to implement those skills if you find a partner who matches your most fundamental characteristics. You don't have to fall victim to fantasies and erroneous beliefs about dating and marriage or believe that mismatches are natural. With the right tools and the right attitude, you can find your perfect partner.

Relationship books tend to fit one of three categories:

-How to develop strong relationship skills

-How to find a partner
-How to have good sex

Perfect Partners speaks to all three issues and uniquely challenges the myth that a great marriage has to be hard work.

We believe in complete honesty. While games may be fun to play, they will almost always lead to disaster. We encourage readers to understand exactly who they are and show them how to find a partner who matches their most essential characteristics. We speak directly to both women and men.

We believe that a great marriage is a more powerful and motivating goal than a winning social life. We place emphasis on marketing and selecting the right partner.

Readers can find partners who match their most essential characteristics. If they put their time and effort into finding the right partner, they won't need <u>Men Are From Mars, Women Are From Venus</u>.

We ask readers to challenge the status quo and put their effort into finding the right partner. They don't have to choose their opposite.

We differentiate between great and good marriages and take the hit-or-miss guesswork out of searching for the right partner.

Our book is positive. It helps readers clearly define who's right for them and teaches them how to find that person. It also addresses the issue of intense competition and the need for exposure to high concentrations of eligible partners.

We bring 30 years of personal and 20 years of professional skills to the subject. Our 16 characteristics are more specific than any list we've seen in any book written thus far and we consider all 16 characteristics to be equally important.

Great sex is a component of a great marriage. We believe that to have great sex you need a partner whose basic sex drive matches yours. We focus on how to find and marry the right partner. In the interest of educating readers, we offer an explicit example of great sex as we have shared it in our marriage.

We're delighted that you've decided to take the plunge and elevate marriage to the high esteem it deserves before it got such a bad name.

We can't stress enough, that, if you follow the process we've articulated in this book, you, too, will find your perfect partner. And what a difference it makes. In an atmosphere of admiration and respect, emotional safety abounds. It's like plugging yourself into electricity. Never have we been so free to become all we are meant to be.

Here's to your audacity to challenge the norm. Thank you for letting us light your way to your own perfect partner.

Fondest wishes and best regards,
Carolyn & Wes Huff

Part I

It's Not True That All Marriages
Take a Lot of Hard Work

1

Why People Marry the Wrong Person

Opposites Attract, But They Shouldn't!

We don't believe that marriage is inherently difficult. We don't believe that the kinds of differences between men and women – gender based differences – are the reason marriages fail. Differences that make a difference are not gender based.

Opposites shouldn't attract, but we all know they do. Because couples with differences that make a difference often marry, and because divorce and unhappy marriages are at an all time high, understanding the reasons they attract and marry could prevent untold heartache and pain. Beyond prevention of unhappiness and divorce, a happy and highly functional marriage liberates the time and energy of partners to devote to other aspects of their lives, like being creative, doing meaningful work, and having fun balanced with satisfying work. And our children need us to break the cycle of what's always been before and model better marriages.

When you choose your mate based on physical chemistry, which most people do, and your idea of who they are isn't who they really are, you and your partner are bound to end up in a marriage with differences that make a difference.

Unfortunately, because people with differences that make a difference attract so often, common belief has it that marriage takes a lot of work. This faulty thinking then goes on to include, since all marriages take a lot of hard work, you must look for someone good enough, realizing that you can't have everything. By the time you realize the serious problems brought about by your differences, you're married. Then, professionals approach marriage from a standpoint of fixing broken marriages with improved relationship skills. Professionals, friends, and relatives tell us we'll never find the perfect person. They say it always looks better elsewhere, but it never really is better. They say no one person can ever provide you with complete companionship, nor with complete need satisfaction. They say no one's perfect. And they say make the best of it, you have to work to make it work. But 50% of our marriages end in divorce, and another 33% are marriages of convenience. We all need to take an honest look at what else is missing in relationships other than interpersonal skills.

Humans aren't perfect, but you can find a partner that's perfect for you. It's possible to have a great marriage. You have to put your effort up front to find the right person, because marrying the wrong person can't be fixed. You can improve your communication and conflict resolution, you can decide to do the things you each like to do separately, but if you're not compatible on differences that make a difference, you can't make yourselves compatible, later. If you have to choose between working continuously at your marriage to achieve peaceful coexistence or spending time and energy to find the right person to have a great marriage, which would you choose? Our goal is to convince you that putting time and energy into the search for the right person offers rewards beyond your greatest expectations.

To begin to persuade you to change your attitude and expectation about what you can have, let's start by looking at the reasons people marry the wrong person. While one or two of the reasons may be carried out by more or less women than men or vice versa, these reasons are not gender based. Both men and women make these mistakes.

Why People Marry the Wrong Person

-Physical chemistry overcomes all sensibility.

-Familiarity – marrying someone just like dear old dad, or mom, or someone else from your past.

-Limited choices.

-One or both partners hide their true self.

-Women believe they have to settle for what they can get because of the belief that all men are afraid of making a commitment.

-Filling in your gaps. Being drawn to someone whose strengths are your perceived weaknesses.

-Rescue fantasies. Not realizing that you don't have to surrender to the prince and the princess fantasy.

-Approval seeking. Basing your choice on the need for approval from others.

-Not realizing you don't have to repeat your parents' pattern.

-Not knowing yourself.

-You didn't know falling in love is a decision.

-Believing all marriages have some degree of mismatch, no other way exists.

-Getting tangled up in the idea of unconditional positive regard or unconditional love.

-Not knowing that the wrong choice is so bad.

Physical chemistry overcomes all sensibility.

Many people believe that physical chemistry is the sign that you belong with someone. Overcome with sexual tension, the person begins a sexual relationship with their prospective partner early in the relationship. Becoming sexual deepens the attachment to someone, so by the time you find out you're not compatible, you've reached a level of attachment that's going to cause a lot of pain if you stay and a lot of pain if you leave.

Wes was so relieved to have a sex partner that he failed to notice the differences between his first wife and him. Meeting someone at the age of 23 who would have a sexual relationship with him released sexual tension stored since adolescence. The torrent of sexual feelings overwhelmed the possibility of thinking about whether they had anything else in common. Wanting to keep his sexual outlet, he tolerated being ridiculed for many of his behaviors, which set the stage for an imbalance of power from the beginning of the marriage. Not only were there major differences between Wes and his first wife, but she used the differences as proof that Wes was a bad person.

While sexual attraction was the overwhelming factor in guiding Wes to marry the wrong person, limited choices, not knowing how bad bad can be, picking someone with whom his parents' would approve, and not knowing who his potential partner really was all played a part.

When you have basic compatibility with

someone on matters that count, physical chemistry will actually increase over time. Natural admiration and affection deepen intimacy. When all you have is physical attraction, that may end the moment the next attractive person comes along.

Familiarity – marrying someone just like dear old dad, or mom, or someone else from your past.

When you're growing up, the behaviors you see demonstrated become connected to what you believe is love. If you witness friendliness, sharing, and respect, you believe that's love. If you see physical and verbal abuse, you believe that's love. If your parents bicker, you believe that's love. Later, you get attracted to people who remind you of what you're used to. This reason is heightened if you have unfinished business with a significant person in your past – like a parent. You'll keep picking people who'll give you the opportunity to master the situation.

One woman with whom Carolyn worked was unhappily married for the third time. As Carolyn listened to her describe her marriages and her partners she heard an all too familiar pattern. This woman was repeatedly marrying men who had most of the relationship problems her father has. Her father had abused her; she'd married one man who had sexually abused their daughter and her playmates and was now married to a man that needed a mother not a wife. He was abusive to her in every way except sexually. She kept marrying men just like her father.

When you marry someone like one of your parents and that parent has wonderful qualities, it's a good thing. But when you're drawn to destructive qualities, it's another story.

To top it off, this woman's daughter is now dating young men that share the same destructive qualities. The pattern is being passed on to the next generation. Several members of this woman's family have similar relationships.

A young man in treatment found himself in one unhappy relationship after another. One day he said to Carolyn, "why do I always end up with mean, bitchy women?" When Carolyn asked him to think about whether the woman he was with reminded him of anyone in his past, he said she reminded him of his mother, who never seemed satisfied with any man. As he described his mother in greater detail to Carolyn, it dawned on him that most of the women he dated demonstrated great hostility toward men. Just like his mother. Without thinking, he'd come to the conclusion that hostility must be love. With that realization he asked, "aren't all women mean and bitchy?" Carolyn's answer was, "of course not." But there are enough that it wasn't difficult for him to reinforce the notion. He was drawn to them and not nice, friendly, warm women. Once he started paying more attention he began to identify the nice ones more and more. Being attentive and conscious about women and how they behave was all it took to change the kind of women he dated.

Something similar happened to Carolyn.

Her parents have an angry tone to their conversations most of the time. Often the hostility conveyed harbored a put down to their partner. They pick on each other and bicker as a general rule. Carolyn and her first husband continued that pattern through most of their marriage. One of Carolyn's children has repeated the pattern in his relationships. Fortunately, her son has the benefit of Carolyn's having brought this pattern to his awareness, and he and his partner actively work at changing their habit of bickering.

As you can imagine, bickering and complaining can undermine trust and love in short order.

It may seem incredible that you can repeatedly stumble upon the same kind of person time after time. How could you possibly keep running into the same circumstance? How can that person be just like the others when he or she didn't appear that way in the beginning? How can you miss the clues? The answer is that many subtle and not so subtle mannerisms and remarks clue us to familiar types of people. We're drawn to them because they're familiar.

Wouldn't it be remarkable if we had so many great marriages around that we could repeat that pattern?

Limited choices.

You can limit your choices in many ways. Competition limits your choices. Looking for a perfect person rather than a perfect partner limits your choices. When you believe that physical attraction is the sign of the right partner you limit your choices. If you believe finding the right marriage partner results from a romantic accident, you limit your choices. Family and friends have their own ideas about suitable mates and their choices for you may fit their agenda more than your needs. The stake they have in their relationship with you influences who they think should be your partner. Following the advice of your friends and family may limit your choices. Only looking in certain places limits your choices. Not knowing the real you limits your choices. Only dating certain types limits your choices. Not dating many people limits your choices.

You have a decidedly decreased chance of finding your perfect partner if you limit your choices.

Wes majored in physics in college. Few women crossed his path because there weren't any female physics majors. He had trouble meeting women to date. To remedy his situation he had to take some courses outside his major so he could enlarge his social group. Even then, only looking on his college campus in a course or two restricted his choice seriously. His fear of not finding a marriage partner was intensified because of his limited search. His lack of practice at dating further limited his choice because of limited experience. All of these factors drove Wes to settle for the best person he could find. And she was not his perfect partner.

To find the right partner for a great marriage you must enlarge your pool of choices to the largest degree possible.

One or both partners hide their true self.

To borrow a term from Zig Ziglar, "over-selling yourself" can only postpone the moment of truth. Hiding your real self, and accommodating to another person's wishes may make you feel safe and in control of the other person's approval of you at the moment, but over the long run, masquerading as someone else isn't safe at all. Maintaining a façade necessitates manipulation and control, and wastes precious energy. Being someone you are not precludes a foundation of trust – you can't trust yourself, and you can't trust what the other person will do if the real you slips out by accident. You certainly can't trust that the other person likes you for yourself. And letting the real you slip out is bound to happen sooner or later.

Mike married a young woman after dating a year and a half. He thought he knew his bride, but didn't. Jennifer was sweet and cooperative, always seeking Mike's opinion, while they dated. He had no idea she hated his work and the hours he spent doing it. He had no idea Jennifer fully expected him to get a regular nine to five job as soon as they married. She expected him to settle into married life as her dad had.

Mike was devastated when he learned what Jennifer expected of him – after the wedding. Within days she started nagging and yelling and manipulating to get him to change. But Mike loved his job and had no intention of changing. Their marriage lasted three months. They're lucky. Many feel trapped and don't leave for years, or spend a lifetime in misery.

Women believe they have to settle for what they can get because of the belief that all men are afraid of making a commitment.

Compounding the problem, most men believe they're supposed to play hard-to-get, so they become what they believe they should be. This paradox exists because we believe it's that way, not because it is that way. Many women settle for whomever they can catch because they believe this is true.

The reason we believe this is learned behavior rather than biologically inborn is that plenty of men exist that aren't afraid of commitment and plenty of men exist that don't play hard-to-get games.

Christie wanted to get married and have a couple of children. At 36 her panic at the prospects of no marriage and children pushed her to the brink of marriage with someone who, after four years together thought they might as well go ahead. At first Christie felt relieved, then she felt deeply disappointed. Christie wanted to marry someone who felt romantic and passionate about marriage to her. Friends, relatives, and her own self-doubt almost had her planning the wedding. She thought she just wanted too much; she thought she was probably selfish to want so much. And there wasn't much time....

Fortunately, Christie's disappointment deepened to the point that she sought help with her dilemma. Coaching from family and friends made her question herself briefly, but no longer gave her any relief from the dread she felt. Christie called off the wedding and made a commitment to therapy and finding the relationship for which she dreamed. She refused to believe all men are the same. She refused to believe men have to be trapped into marriage because none of them really want to marry.

Filling in your gaps. Being drawn to someone whose strengths are your perceived weaknesses.

Many of us end up in a relationship with someone who fills in our gaps. If you're messy and disorganized, you're drawn to a neat person. If you're a perfectionist about neatness, you pick someone more relaxed about being neat. These traits influence other things, too, like how you handle money, and whether you balance your checkbook. You look for balance from your partner rather than within yourself. Unfortunately, the very traits you're grateful to your partner for having initially are usually the things that end up making you crazy over time.

We surveyed local Parents Without Partners groups and many of them stated they were looking for skills in their partners that they didn't have. Some of the tasks they wanted new partners to be able to do were handy-man work, good cooking, and making more money. These are common examples of tasks people look for in a partner that they themselves could do. Or hire someone to do. Don't select a marriage partner because they can do tasks you can't do – to fill in your gaps. Choose a marriage partner similar to you and either learn to do the task yourself or hire someone.

Tony handled money carefully, balancing his budget and saving for the future. Jessica never knew how much of her paycheck she'd spent; she overdrew her bank account regularly. Tony was extremely neat; he always helped with the household chores. Jessica had never known a man that was so helpful. And he always had the money he needed for whatever he wanted to do. She felt safe and cared for. Tony felt admired for his neatness and careful financial planning. He felt protective toward and needed by Jessica.

Jessica didn't realize until a few years into the marriage that Tony's neatness was paranoia about germs and gaining the approval of his parents. His need for neatness was unrealistic and rigid – impossible with which to live. His careful financial planning felt stingy to her within months. Tony absorbed himself in the details of life, which ended up distracting him from intimacy and fun. Because Tony's neat and miserly behaviors helped him manage tremendous anxiety about life and being accepted, relaxing his standards was impossible. Jessica felt miserable. Tony criticized her constantly because he couldn't tolerate any deviation from his way of handling life's tasks. And he despised what he finally saw as childishness and irresponsibility in his wife.

Understand the differences aren't the problem, but making the other person into the bad guy is. Some differences make a difference and it's wrong to expect others to become you. There are many "right" ways to do things. The point is to match yourself with someone that already does things similar to you so you don't feel like you have to fight to the finish to make the other person act and think and feel just like you.

Rescue fantasies. Not realizing that you don't have to surrender to the prince and the princess fantasy.

Some people believe that the woman should wait to be swept of her feet by a man who acts like a prince. What's good about the prince and princess theory is the implication that someone perfect exists for everyone. What's bad is sitting back and waiting. Another problem is that, even if someone comes along who looks like a prince, no guarantees exist that you'll match this particular prince.

At 38 Darlene was dating a man who came on to her like the prince she awaited. The first six months of their relationship Darlene could do no wrong. She believed she'd finally found her prince. She did have some lurking hesitation because she'd been with other charming men who, later into their relationship, turned into men who wanted everything their way. Wooed by his charm and attention, showered with affection, each time Darlene believed this man was the perfect partner. Before Vince, all of the men Darlene dated showed their true colors over time. Eventually they all became emotionally, mentally, and some, physically abusive. Each time, Darlene broke off the relationship with much pain and hopelessness. Each time Darlene went back for more. Because she didn't

modify her approach to finding a marriage partner, because she didn't alter her pattern of waiting to be saved by her prince, at 38 Darlene kept
getting stuck with the same kind of man repeatedly. She didn't realize to find a different kind of
man she needed to look in places where she'd
never looked; she didn't realize she needed to
actively look, not sit back and wait. Quickly, her
instinct that Vince is the same kind of man
proved to be accurate.

More women than men wait to be rescued.
More men than women see themselves as res-
cuers. Being rescued and rescuing always imply
someone's dependence. When both partners are
competent adults, neither needs to be rescued
nor to be seen as the rescuer.

**Approval seeking. Basing your choice on the
need for approval from others.**

As children we're dependent upon our parents
for survival. We're exquisitely vulnerable, easily
controlled. Most of us do whatever we need to
do to gain our parent's approval. If your parents
valued you as an individual and respected your
feelings and thoughts when you were a child,
you grew up having a high regard for yourself,
trusting your perceptions and ability to figure
things out. You learn to think for yourself.
Because you trust yourself, you have the ability
to check within for approval. If your parents
used shame and humiliation to control your
behavior, disregarded your feelings and
thoughts, and insisted you act and think their
way, you grew up afraid to trust yourself and

your perceptions. And you can't think for yourself. Since you don't trust yourself, you have to
check with others for approval.

If you need approval from others, you'll
pick the person others believe you should
marry not necessarily the right partner for you.

Carolyn's parents disapproved of every
boy she dated until she dated her first husband.
Her first boyfriends were always from the wrong
side of town in her parents' eyes. They breathed
a sigh of relief when she began to date someone
they believed came from the right kind of family, someone from the right part of town. Carolyn
has no way of knowing how a marriage with any
of those first young men she dated would have
turned out, but she knows how her first marriage turned out. Being from the right side of
town and the right kind of family is no guarantee you match, and no guarantee the man or
woman has achieved maturity. Carolyn's parents measured this young man's fitness on
superficial qualities; they had no idea he had a
problem drinking; they had no idea he taught
Carolyn to drink and smoke; they had no idea
he taught her to drive without a license. All of
which is a blatant display of disregard for social
rules and responsibility. And Carolyn didn't
know any better. Young and inexperienced, she
only knew she'd finally gained her parents'
approval.

**Not realizing you don't have to repeat your
parents' pattern.**

In most areas of life, truly successful people

think for themselves. When you live your life without thinking about the choices you have or automatically do what your parents have done, you're living without thinking about what you're doing – you're living unconsciously and unaware. If your parents' choice of mate resulted in a great marriage, you're home free imitating your parents. But picking your perfect partner for marriage doesn't usually happen to people who don't think for themselves. And none of us are clones of our parents.

Parents don't always obviously disapprove of a prospective partner. Your parents' pattern of raising you may have instilled the belief that you must always act and think like them. By the time you get into dating and picking a marriage partner, you may imitate your parents so closely you don't realize you're picking a partner based on their approval.

There's no place like an abusive, violent childhood home that more obviously illustrates how destructive blind imitation can be.

His father beat John many times. His father regularly beat his mother. As a child, John survived by submitting to his father's demands, but by the time he went into the world on his own he had stuffed a lot of rage. Without realizing, he had identified with the aggressor, and to handle his rage and gain a sense of power, he joined the Marines, which was a positive channel for the feelings he has. When he married, he picked a partner just like mom; and he treated his wife and children just like dad had treated his wife and children, which was destructive.

Another example is Susan. Susan's mother took one year off between graduating from college and returning to graduate school. Her mother lived with a boyfriend during graduate school and married that boyfriend. She married him even though they were incompatible. Susan's mother didn't really like the man she married and over time her resentment grew. Eventually, her husband's desire for an active and robust sex life turned into torture for her. For a while she used sex to control his behavior. Finally she was so angry all of the time, she called him a rapist.

Susan's daughter, Elizabeth, never separated psychologically (never learned to think and feel for herself) from her mother, so her life replicates her mother's closely. Elizabeth took a year off after graduating from college before returning to graduate school. She dates men who have little in common with her. As is often the case, patterns and themes passed on from generation to generation, find behaviors becoming more distilled; Elizabeth dated a real rapist. Elizabeth handled conflict the same as her mother; she avoided it as much as possible. She acted out her mother's anger at her father, and believed her mother's interpretation of her father's behavior without question. Since conflict was taboo, she hated her father even more for what she saw as his causing so much conflict because he was a bad person. One of the ways she coped with her rage toward her father after all attempts to shame and control him failed, was to cut off emotionally from him entirely. Since she has refused to finish her unfinished business with her father directly, she's compelled to master the situation in another relationship. Now she's in a live-in relationship, just like her mother's pattern, with a man just like her father.

Not knowing yourself.

Knowing yourself takes time, life experiences, and opportunity. Being alive long enough takes care of time and experience; opportunity takes an environment that allows you to express your thoughts and feelings and tolerates your decision-making and mistakes.

If you don't know yourself, how can you know what you want or what matches another person?

Carolyn had a serious problem that represents an issue many women experience. You don't know what you think, what you like, what you believe, and you don't know how you feel (men have trouble knowing they feel tender and loving and that those feelings aren't emasculating, women have the most trouble connecting with their anger and that anger doesn't automatically kill). Like most women, Carolyn's life revolved around taking care of others, which made knowing what they wanted much more important than what she wanted or knew or believed. She regularly held back feelings – so called negative feelings, like anger and sorrow. She left the home of her parents and went directly into marriage without a pause to find out who she was. Carolyn spent thirty years in three relationships, all of which were the wrong partner for her. Until she'd spent time by her-self, she had no opportunity to get to know her-self. Minus the distractions of a relationship, she connected with her own self.

You didn't know falling in love is a decision – a choice.

Contrary to what many people believe, love is behavior not a feeling. You act loving toward someone or something. Affection, admiration, gratitude, sexual attraction, respect, happiness, joy, commitment, loyalty are feelings associated with loving actions. Fear can even trick people into believing they love someone. The fear is associated with dependency, loss, rejection, or abandonment.

If you don't believe love is a way to behave, a choice, you're most likely mixing up the feelings you're having with fear and a belief that you have no control over how you feel or act toward someone.

Trisha fought with her boyfriend con-stantly. She felt suicidal on several occasions because of their fights. Joe was nineteen and Trisha, 26. Each week in therapy she would lament the latest events of her relationship with Joe. In the last twelve months of their 14-month relationship, Joe had been sick or recovering from surgery most of the time. Trisha's rela-tionship with Joe revolved around taking care of his needs. A few times Trisha sought solace from Joe, but he was too busy with himself to allow Trisha some give and take. He repeatedly canceled plans at the last moment. Trisha felt disappointed all of the time. In order to get her needs met, Trisha competed with Joe for who needed taken care of. In therapy she sobbed. In middle-of-the- night phone calls, she sobbed and threatened suicide. On one occasion she cut herself with a knife in a suicidal gesture.

When Carolyn explored what was happening in Trisha's relationship with Joe, all Trisha could do was wail, "but I love him."

Sorry folks. The feelings here are fear, desperation, panic, dependency, not love.

Believing all marriages have some degree of mismatch, no other way exists.

When you believe something – like anyone can have wealth if they want it – you actually set up the exact circumstances for the outcome you expect. If you believe finding the perfect mate is impossible, it will be. If you believe life doesn't have to be the way someone else says life has to be, you'll have more options for directing your own life, getting the outcome you want. Getting what you want depends on a questioning, challenging mind and determination to seek what you want. You have to avoid blindly accepting what's always come before. Behaving like others just because most do is a poor reason for doing something. Behaving like others, even when their behavior has a bad outcome is especially self-defeating. And not trying something new just because that action has never been done before is equally limiting.

Anne's live-in boyfriend of four years just broke off their relationship. She stayed in the relationship this long, not because she believed this man was her perfect partner, but because she'd invested so much. She believed men needed catching and that all marriages take hard work. Time was running out (she was 36 years old) and she thought he'd be good enough. After all, she'd already hung in there this long. And if all men are alike, she may as well say or do whatever it takes to catch this one. This is the fourth significant relationship she's been in that ended because she wanted to get married and have children and her boyfriend didn't want a commitment. Hurting, she wanted to understand. It didn't take long to discover that Anne believed all men were alike. She reinforced that belief by only looking in one place for potential partners, which caused her to run into the same kind of man over and over.

Fred wanted to know how to manage his wife. He believed all women were alike and the key to a happy marriage was learning how to manage your wife's behavior. We find it hard to believe that any man or woman wants to be managed.

Fred relates to others as though they were an extension of him. It has never occurred to him that marriage is two people that think and feel for themselves. Since he believes all women are alike (he's heard it a hundred times), it has never occurred to him to find someone with whom he matches on certain qualities so he won't have to manage them or himself.

Getting tangled up in the idea of unconditional positive regard or unconditional love.

Years ago a wonderful psychologist, Carl Rogers, developed the notion of unconditional positive regard. Unconditional positive regard is the act of respect. Rogers believed unconditional positive regard was the element necessary in our early relationships that allows us to develop as our true selves. This is a wonderful concept and it has helped us understand that children need to be treated as human beings with respect. They are little people that don't know much yet, not pets. Please notice that he doesn't call unconditional positive regard unconditional permissiveness.

Unfortunately, many people have misinterpreted this concept to mean tolerance for someone's behavior – unconditional permissiveness – no matter how they act. Unconditional permissiveness is a serious distortion of what Dr. Rogers meant. Allowing ourselves to be treated in harmful ways is destructive. Allowing ourselves to behave any way we want, expecting unconditional positive regard, is ridiculous.

Unconditional positive regard means interacting with other people with an attitude of respect. Unconditional positive regard doesn't mean accepting and approving any kind of behavior no matter how destructive. Unconditional positive regard means taking the ridicule, shame, humiliation, mockery, and self-righteousness out of your interactions. Ruthlessly murdering another person because you're drunk or from a deprived background are not excuses for your behavior. Knowing you were drunk or deprived as a child is information for understanding the behavior – maybe in the future we can apply the information to raising children so we can prevent more of this behavior. But using the information to allow murder is inappropriate.

Tolerating, justifying, and rationalizing unacceptable behavior in a relationship – unconditional permissiveness – is self-destructive.

Jane married a man who demanded that everything be done his way. He ran around with other women – she contracted herpes from him after their marriage. He refused to leave an impossible work situation for years. His behavior and demands tortured Jane and the children, but Jane stayed. She tried to commit suicide on several occasions, but she stayed. Jane justified Dan's behavior by recognizing that his traumatic childhood left him with destructive ways of relating to others. His mother committed suicide when he was three years old and he couldn't help himself. He needed her. She rationalized staying by believing her relationship with him would repair the damage. She nearly lost her own life doing so. Jane sees being a wife as having no needs of her own, only catering to the needs of the other person.

The problem about unconditional permissiveness is not only not getting your needs met, but depriving the other person of a reality check on their behavior. By protecting them from the natural consequences of their behavior, they never have to look at what they do and how they act. In essence, not exposing them to natural consequences deprives them of an opportunity to change for the better. It's also an unspoken message that the person acting in a destructive way isn't capable of improving their behavior. That's rarely true.

The distortion of unconditional positive regard to unconditional permissiveness is at the root of most social problems in our culture today. It's a seriously destructive distortion of a benevolent and affirming idea. The distortion ruins lives, ruins marriages, and ruins families.

Not knowing that the wrong choice is so bad.

When you're young and inexperienced you don't always believe what happens to others can also happen to you. For a variety of reasons, you believe you're impervious to the things that harm others and believe bad things won't happen to you. You can go into relationships believing you won't repeat the same mistakes you've seen so many others make. When you add, believing all marriages take a lot of work, to the rest of your beliefs, you increase the odds of marrying the wrong person.

Divorce on demand and living together as options can compound the problems of this thinking, because they're seen as an escape hatch. Divorce and living together are options, and divorce is sometimes better than any alternative, but divorce and splitting after living together are very painful. Divorce and ending a live-in relationship are often more painful than the death of someone close. People just don't realize. Just because you have the option doesn't make it painless or harmless. We should maintain the option of divorce. No individual should be trapped in a marriage to someone to whom they don't want to be married. People aren't possessions. But we must make a greater effort to prevent divorce. Divorce always hurts everyone.

All of the reasons people marry the wrong person boil down to reacting to life rather than directing your life. You have nothing to lose, except powerlessness and poor outcomes, by taking charge of your life. You have nothing to lose by thinking and acting for yourself and you have a great marriage to gain.

To some degree, in every example we've given you, the people involved just didn't realize how bad a bad marriage can be. Don't let that happen to you.

2

Not So Perfect

The Land Mines of Marriage
With the Wrong Partner

This book is meant to be an optimistic celebration of what's possible: making your hopes and dreams for a great marriage come true. But being brutally honest about what happens in a marriage to the wrong partner is part of the motivation to avert a painful disaster. Marriage to the wrong partner is the loneliest place of all.

Our intention is to strip away your innocence about bad marriages. If you've been there, you already know. Having been there, some of us still proceed to get into another bad relationship. Without having been there, it's particularly difficult to know what you're getting yourself into. Most people don't believe it can happen to them.

Marriage isn't inherently bad and a lot of hard work. But marriage to the wrong partner is horrendous and a lot of hard work just to limp along. Understand: bad can really be bad in a marriage to the wrong partner. The constant stress of managing differences drives marriages toward divorce and leads to problems such as stress-related illness, emotional turmoil, poor self-esteem, diminished self-confidence, work problems, and addiction. The children of these marriages suffer from sibling jealousy, insecurity, nightmares, school difficulties, drug use, and later, poor relationships of their own.

Most people in bad marriages are ambivalent about whether to stay or to leave. Most people want their marriage to be okay so much – most wish everything will turn out alright intensively – that they trap themselves into ambivalence, which is far worse than ending the wrong marriage. Not being in your marriage, not being out of your marriage is unbearable.

Inertia and fear of the unknown constrain you into the same old behaviors, that can't help but deliver you to the same bad or mediocre marriages as everyone else. Facing the potential injury from exploded land mines can help you decide to choose the right partner. And deciding to marry the right partner is the first step to doing it.

To avoid deepening the trouble of the wrong relationship into stress, emotional pain, and unhappiness for an entire family, stop and consider some new ideas.

Here's the next piece of information with

which to motivate yourself to avoid what doesn't have to be, and actively, intentionally pursue what you can have – a great marriage. No amount of wishful thinking will work. You must do this on purpose.

In general, the outcome of marrying someone whose differences make a difference results in poor, or at best, mediocre marriages.

Poor Marriages

We define a poor marriage as a marriage with the presence of any type of abuse – physical, emotional, or verbal. The partners of a poor marriage have low compatibility on core issues – differences that make a difference – and poor relationship skills. Not only are they different on important issues, but at least one partner blames the other for not being the way they want them to be and believes their way is the best and the only way. Basic respect for others is missing in at least one partner of a poor marriage. Neither partner gets their needs met.

Marriages of Convenience

A mediocre marriage – a marriage of convenience – is a marriage in which the partners get along in terms of peaceful coexistence – most often separating their lives to a great extent. They have a healthy respect for others and, in general, have good relationship skills making incompatibility less destructive. These partners have taken the noble endeavor of tolerating differences to heart. But they have less intimacy, if any, to keep the peace and they participate in separate activities, thereby depriving themselves of the deepening of their bond. They stay in the marriage because of convenience and the idea that it could be worse. Some stay because they believe their duty and commitment means stay no matter what. With their best relationship skills, each partner gets their needs met only part of the time and largely separate from the other.

An energized and nurturing connection based on attraction, admiration, and deeply liking your partner is absent in both poor marriages and marriages of convenience.

Statistics show that 83% of all marriages are either poor or marriages of convenience. Unfortunately, if either partner loses in a marriage, both partners lose.

What Mires Marriage in Ambivalence and Puts It On the Divorce Block?

Mainly, it's exhaustion and pain from the constant strain of managing differences. The kinds of differences, the degree of difference, as well as, the methods a couple uses to manage their differences, spells out making it or not. And making it is in a matter of degrees from peaceful coexistence and parallel play to an energized, great marriage, with a vitality that fuels itself.

A recent survey conducted by Good Housekeeping magazine reports that 70% of married men cheat on their wives. That certainly makes infidelity high on the list of problems.

We see infidelity as a symptom of something that's wrong. Either the marriage is riddled with incompatibility or is crippled with poor relationship skills. Infidelity contributes to lack of trust, which you'll see at the top of the Ladies' Home Journal list below. Or it may be as a result of turning to someone outside the marriage for solace.

Because infidelity is a symptom, you can avoid it in your marriage by attending to the causes. Marry the right partner. Someone that has a high degree of compatibility with you on the 16 differences that make a difference and someone that has matured enough to thrive in marriage.

The Land Mines

The Ladies' Home Journal has featured a column about marriage for fifty years called Can This Marriage Be Saved? It's billed the "most popular, most enduring Women's Magazine feature in the world." This column identifies seven underlying areas causing marital distress, that remain fundamentally the same from generation to generation, no matter what the specifics are from marriage to marriage. These tasks are all things that help or hinder managing differences. They are basically relationship skills or skills of daily living. And the column directs its efforts to mending broken relationships by improving relationship skills.

-Trust
-Poor Communication
-Poor Management of Anger
-Power Struggles
-Money Management
-Problems with Sexual Intimacy
-Outside Pressures from Work, Family
   and Friends

We Would Add
-Differences That Make a Difference
   Resulting in Endless Negotiation and a
   Win-Lose or a Lose-Lose Relationship

Let's look at each category.

Trust

You need to be able to rely on yourself and others. Lack of trust undermines intimacy. You can't trust a partner that has extramarital affairs. You can't trust a partner that shames or humiliates you, and even more so, in front of others. You can't trust a partner that assigns blame to you for every difficulty or disagreement in the marriage. You can't trust a partner that puts you down because your opinion about certain topics differs from theirs. You can't trust a partner who tries to talk you out of your feelings or diminishes your credibility. You can't trust a partner that keeps secrets or hides their real self from you. You can't trust a partner that criticizes you for the way you think, feel, and do things in life. You can't trust a partner that complains to others about you behind your back. You can't trust a partner that doesn't follow through on their promises or who won't carry their fair share of the work and fun of marriage.

Lack of trust between partners undermines any possibility of a great marriage.

When you don't trust yourself, it's hard to trust others even when they're trustworthy. And if you don't trust yourself, how can anyone else trust you? When you can't trust your partner, how can you trust them with your most private feelings and thoughts – intimacy? Lack of trust causes you to look outside your marriage for emotional safety, validation, support, and maybe even sex. Or worse, it causes you to wall yourself off from others and the ability to confide in someone. When trust is absent, marriage isn't marriage; it's a cold war at best.

Distrust can come from past experiences and be transferred to your present circumstances. But distrust most often comes from having differences that make a difference. When someone handles money differently than you do, how can you trust each other if your partner continuously manages money in a way that makes you anxious? If one of the most important ways you feel loved is with sexual expression and making love, how can you trust a partner that has a low sex drive? If holding hands and frequent hugs and kisses are a major part of demonstrations of affection and admiration for you, how can you trust someone that cringes when you try to hold hands in public? If you love to spend the weekend quietly at home reading and listening to music, how can you trust your partner to help you satisfy your needs if he or she likes to spend their weekends in numerous social activities with the more participants the better?

A major source of distrust is adultery.

Diane felt betrayed when she learned that Doug was having an affair. They were working on issues of trust and attempting to repair their marriage when Diane learned that Doug's affair wasn't the first. When Diane realized that Doug was involved in extramarital affairs since the beginning of their marriage, seven years ago, she simply couldn't go on in the marriage. And when he blamed the affairs on Diane, because she wouldn't give him enough sex, she initially believed that she was the cause of his behavior. Diane began to doubt herself. She divorced Doug, but the idea that she was to blame was a constant drain on her feelings about herself. Diane spent several years repairing the damage to her self-esteem and self-confidence. Fortunately she did repair the damage, but it took her several years to trust herself and men enough to begin dating again.

Tom and Suzanne escalated toward almost constant conflict. Their differences permeated their lives. They couldn't agree on how often to have sex, or how to handle money, or how to raise the children. Their interests led them in different directions. The destruction of their marriage escalated to destruction of Tom's relationship with his daughter. Suzanne had begun to complain about Tom to their daughter. She blamed and accused him of every problem and fault of their marriage. Tom tried to get them into counseling, but Suzanne wouldn't go. He tried to get Suzanne to read some books and address their problems. But Suzanne didn't believe she had anything to do with their problems. Suzanne believed they were more than just different. Tom wouldn't do whatever she wanted, the way she wanted, so he was bad and evil. She was sexually inhibited, so, in her eyes, Tom's enjoyment of sex was unnatural, even perverted. For many years of their marriage, and their daughter's life, Suzanne criticized and complained to their daughter about her father.

The result of this disaster was divorce. But not until a father's relationship with his daughter had been destroyed, possibly forever.

Tom's daughter believes any show of interest in her life or activities on her father's part are an attempt to control her. When he attempted to set limits for her as a child, her mother intervened to stop him and to give their daughter her way. His daughter interpreted certain behaviors during her childhood as bad and evil, not merely relaxation and comfort in his own home.

For instance, Tom liked to sit around and watch TV in a tee shirt. The only TV was in the living room. The curtains on the windows only partially covered the windows. Years later, when his new wife bought him boxer shorts, he said, "Boy, I sure wish I'd known how comfortable these were before. It might have saved me from all the criticism about running around in the buff." Tom's efforts at comfort in his home would have been interpreted in most households as normal relaxation. Most wives would have helped their husband have the most comfort possible. Most wives would have suggested more comfortable clothing and put more private curtains on the windows. But because of Suzanne's interpretation of the behaviors, their daughter and she treated the behaviors as perverted. Because Suzanne didn't like Tom and believed that he was bad because he didn't do everything her way, the real circumstances were misinterpreted. Most wives would have never involved a child in the destructive interpretations just to justify their behavior and feelings. Most parents know better than to confide marital secrets to their children. But Tom didn't have most wives. He had a wife with serious differences and very poor marital skills.

The destruction of their relationship is seriously troubling to Tom, but the worst destruction of all has been to his daughter. Her mother has modeled choosing the wrong marriage partner and then blaming him for their differences. Her mother took away any ability for her daughter to trust her father, so anything he might have to offer her is discredited. She transfers her distrust of men to the partners she dates. Her father demonstrates a stable maturity in his life and is effective in most things he does, but his daughter learned to distrust the good qualities along with the so-called bad qualities. This young woman has been deprived of a positive relationship with her father and the model of a mature marital relationship so her mother could maintain the position that she's wonderful and dad is awful. Even now, several years after the divorce, Suzanne refuses to own her piece of the misery. She refuses to guide her daughter into a more realistic and favorable picture of Tom. Tom can't repair the damage because his daughter has cut off any relationship with him. The opportunity to see her father in a more honest light, happy in a marriage with a new partner lost because of her emotional cutoff from her father. She hasn't spoken a civil word or allowed any communication with her father for more than two years.

Suzanne's solution is that Tom goes to therapy because he's disturbed. She keeps forgetting that he doesn't have any trouble going to therapy at all. She forgets that she is the one that is afraid of therapy and won't go. Suzanne's the one that won't read a book that might shine some light on her problems. Five years after their divorce Suzanne and her daughter maintain that Tom is the only problem in their life.

Interesting to note is that his daughter's cutoff didn't happen until another woman came into Tom's life with which he found a high level of compatibility – two years after her parents divorced. As his daughter had more exposure to him in a happy and compatible marriage, she became more threatened. Finally, she couldn't tolerate any examination of the possibility that he wasn't the problem. And she cut off all contact. It would be interesting to know how many generations these distorted beliefs will be passed down. The bad marriage between Tom and Suzanne didn't just end with their divorce.

Poor Communication

How can you satisfy your partner's needs if they never tell you what their needs are? How can you communicate clearly when what your partner is saying is inflammatory to you? How can you communicate affection, respect, and admiration to your partner when you disagree on basic values and views of the world? How can you support someone emotionally when what he or she is doing is seriously contrary to what you believe?

Respectful toleration of differences is a valuable aspect of mature function in the world. Stretching yourself by keeping an open mind and exposing yourself to new ideas is useful to maintain civil communities and to your own growth. But marital partners live in too intense a relationship to ask their values to be in question everyday. When your values are in question all of the time, you only have time and energy to debate and defend your position. You only have time and energy to talk yourself into accepting your partner the way they are and to try to call back the affection and attraction through all of the mixed emotions. Marriage partners need to provide a safe haven for themselves and their partner. They need to raise their children in a physically and emotionally safe and predictable environment. They need that stability and the encouragement and emotional support to conquer other challenges in life.

There is no question that good communication can help partners that disagree do so in a respectful and friendly way. But even good communication cannot make you compatible with your partner if you have different values. And poor communication adds salt to the wound.

Poor communication can be related to poor delivery or reception of messages, and/or related to your attitude toward others. People that communicate indirectly don't get their messages across often. People that receive messages through the filter of a painful past or a distorted past, rarely receive the real and intended message. If your attitude is win-win and you're determined to understand your partner, your attitude of respect will enhance your communication. Without an attitude of win-win and a desire to understand and be understood, communication will seriously limit your marriage to poor, or at best, mediocre.

Conflict created by marriage to a person that has little compatibility with you on important issues tests communication skills to their maximum. Good communication can save a marriage from being abusive. Poor communication usually escalates conflict into the abusive range.

Tonya and Robert had a marriage filled with conflict. They disagreed often and any attempts Tonya made to clarify their communication met with personal attacks by Robert. He would say things like, "aren't you ever satisfied?" Or, "you are the most selfish person I've ever met in my life. All you want is to satisfy yourself. You never think about me or the children." Robert was marginally adequate to handle everyday life. The responsibilities of marriage and fatherhood had taxed him beyond his capacity to function. Feeling badly about himself, he used every opportunity to make sure others thought he was smart and right. Robert argued defensively, to the death, over everything. In therapy he even argued against his own points when Carolyn reflected back to him what he'd said. Argument and opposition was his automatic response to whatever anyone else said. Every request from his wife felt like an unreasonable demand. Robert disregards everything Tonya says to him or others, discounting her opinions. In therapy one day, when Robert didn't like what Carolyn had to say about their marriage, Robert said, "you don't have a single bit of evidence to make your assessment of what is happening in our marriage." So Carolyn asked, "does that mean that not a single thing your wife has told me about your marriage over the last six months is true? Does that mean nothing she tells me is true?" He didn't know what to say. When Carolyn asked, "doesn't anything your wife has to say have merit", he still didn't know what to say.

This couple's marriage is rapidly escalating to divorce. Carolyn hopes they'll end the marriage before someone gets hurt physically.

No possibility exists to end the marriage before emotional damage occurs; Tonya and the three children in the home have trouble sleeping, eating, staying well, and going to school and to work, already. Robert may seem to be the only survivor, but he's harming himself along with his mate and children every time he demeans himself with his destructive communication and behavior.

Tanya and Robert provide an example of actively destructive communication, but less obvious and more passive forms of poor communication exist, that are also destructive over time. When a partner doesn't speak up and let you know what they think and feel, they have poor communication. You can't solve a problem if all you ever do is complain to a third party about something going on in your marriage. Again, notice that the poor communication only contributes to increasing their incompatibility. If they didn't have important core differences, their poor communication wouldn't be such a problem.

Poor Management of Anger

Anger is the natural result of displeasure. Anger is a wake up call that something is wrong. If we notice our anger, it can help us decide what is in our best interest to do. If we notice we're angry most of the time, or never, that in itself, offers us important information.

Just like communication, anger can be

handled for better or for worse. And just like communication, without serious differences, anger wouldn't be an over-riding element in your marriage. Mismanagement of anger adds another layer of discontent. Mismanagement of anger comes in all kinds of different packages.

Jill and Andy had all the appearances of a successful marriage. No one ever heard them disagree. There was no fighting in the household. But Jill and Andy had unresolved conflicts, which escalated into bitter resentment over time. Their style of managing differences and anger resulted in numbing themselves to many of their feelings, including affection, happiness, and joy. Avoiding the recognition and expression of their anger didn't resolve their conflicts, however. Anger that has been stuffed inside over a long period of time has a habit of spewing forth at the most inopportune times. For Jill and Andy, the day came when the anger could be contained no more. Jill screamed, " I hate you. All you ever do is think about yourself. All you ever want is sex. Well I hate having sex with you. You've ruined sex for me. Leave me alone," while she threw anything she could get her hands on. She threw personal attacks and she threw furniture. The anger was postponed, but not gone. When the anger finally came, it ended the marriage.

Anne and Steve didn't have any problem expressing their anger. They had plenty of disagreements so their life was filled with loud, verbal conflict. The only problem was that anger permeated their lives and left little time for any fun. Their friends had difficulty exposing themselves to the constant conflict because it was such a negative drain. The personal attacks contained in their angry interactions finally wore their respect and admiration for each other thin and eventually eroded the positive they once enjoyed about each other. Anne didn't like Steve's drinking. When he drank, Anne would say things like, "you're never there for me. I can't talk to you about anything because you've been drinking." Steve would reply, "well if you weren't such a bitch I wouldn't have anything to drink about." On another occasion Steve said, "if you weren't so fat, I wouldn't drink, because there'd be someone worth coming home to." There were such differences in some core values they held that the passion they had for each other couldn't win over the differences. After hurling such hurtful accusations at one another, how could anyone find the love again?

Meg solved her problem with anger at her father with an emotional cutoff. One-day Meg's dad was alerted to some new information about something that bothered Meg about her relationship with him. When her dad was trying to clarify how he felt and what he thought about something he thought Meg had misinterpreted, Meg screamed, "you're a lying bastard. I never want to see or speak to you again. Leave me alone. You're not allowed to speak to me or think of me ever again." She refused to have any sort of communication with him at all, thereby saving herself from the anger (and loving feelings) she felt toward him. The biggest problem is that since the anger is unresolved it replays itself over and over in her other relationships with men. The choice to manage her anger with a cutoff saddles Meg with the need to resolve her feelings and expectations in other relationships. People are driven to master difficult situations so, without realizing it, Meg has relegated herself to what's called a repetition compulsion. She will find herself in similar situations over and over again, with repeated opportunities to master the developmental task she must master in order to be free to live her life happily.

When you have differences in your values, not only will the big differences make you angry, but the small, everyday nuisances will also make you angry. The more differences that make a difference you have with your partner, the better you'll need to be at managing your anger.

Power Struggles

We recently did a survey of singles, asking them questions regarding their thoughts and feelings about relationships and marriage. One question asked: What kinds of things happened because of your bad marriage? A wide range of answers were given, from financial problems, emotional and physical stress, low self-esteem, decreased self-confidence, diminished trust in others, unhappy children, assault and battery, lost home, adultery, substance abuse and addiction, guilty feelings, suicide attempts, depression, and divorce, divorce, divorce.

All of the problems listed here can be the result of all of the causes of divorce we've listed. You can count on power struggles to contribute heavily to every awful result listed in these respondents' answers.

Current thought is that differences are bound to occur in every marriage and therefore the key to successful maneuvering around such obstacles is to learn to accept your partner and what they believe. They say you don't have to agree, but you must stop competing, criticizing, and blaming. For some things in life like what kind of ice cream you like, or whether you believe ice cream is healthy for you at all, we agree. Stop forcing your ideas on others. Inform them of your ideas, and then let them live the way they want. Hundreds of life's problems can be handled that way. You can stop controlling everyone else's every move, thought and idea, and let go. It's a wonderful feeling to be only responsible for you and let others decide how to live for them.

The problem with this idea in marriage is that differences in your deepest values and beliefs are a set up for a power struggle because of the very nature of your need to live with integrity. You hold some ideas that are simply at the root of what you believe. If you choose to survive in a marriage with differences that make a difference, you will either live separate lives, harboring, at minimum, suspicion of your mate's different beliefs. Or, at worst, with conflict of the worst kind: conflict over your values and beliefs that either you or your mate must relinquish to maintain harmony. And harmony and peace are vital elements of a functional marriage and home. Differences that make a difference challenge your or your partner's integrity and force your children to choose loyalty along with ideals and values. But living without integrity evokes despair. You must fight to the end for your values and principles.

Power struggles in relationships are a set up to win or lose. But if either partner in a marriage loses, both lose. Do you want to be in a marriage where you are guaranteed to lose at least half of the time? Do you want to spend your time and energy on winning or losing every life task? Do you want to spend your time and energy on making sure everyone else lives the way you believe is the right way? If you do, you'll have little time left for anything else. Marriage isn't a competition.

Most people think of the bread-winning male of our past traditional marriages as the controllers of marriages and families. But women have done their own share of controlling their men.

Jean doesn't like sex very much. Sex a few times a year, if any, would be enough for her. Because Jean only favors Paul with sex if everything goes her way, he comes home from work, turns over his paycheck to her to control, submits to her passive discipline of his children, and does just about anything she says to not rock the boat. One behavior out of line would be reason to cut off sex for many days or even weeks.

Rachel uses put downs and directly hurtful comments about Don in front of their friends and children to control Don's behavior. When Don incurs her wrath, he can expect direct, hurtful name-calling. Once she said, in front of friends, "Oh, he's tried to start a business before; he doesn't know what he's doing." Don can't keep up with Rachel verbally. Any attempt at verbal debate results in his loss. Don has learned if he is to ever have control he must win it passively, indirectly. His doing so was what brought them to therapy.

Rachel's complaint was "he won't talk to me about anything." And Rachel was right. Carolyn couldn't count how many times she asked Don how he felt or what he thought that he wouldn't answer at all or would say a one-word answer giving no information at all. Carolyn would say, "how was your week?" Don would reply, "fine." If she said catch me up on what's going on, he'd look at her, smile, and shrug his shoulders. There's one way to keep someone from launching attacks at you and that is to never give them anything to aim their ammunition toward. Don regained some control in his marriage by withdrawing and giving as little information as possible. His way of repaying his mate for her verbal slights was to forget to do something important. His style of gaining some sense of control was passive-aggressive.

Power struggles come in all shapes and sizes. Power struggles in competitive sports can be challenging and fun. Power struggles in marriage doom you to a bad marriage.

Money Management

Money is never just money. Earning, spending, and saving money has many hidden agendas attached like, safety, security, fun, power, control, approval, competence, self-esteem, accomplishment, independence, personal values, excitement, risk. Money can be used as a weapon to punish your mate. Because money is never just money, it's a magnet for problems in marriage. Money means different things to different people and its place in our lives is so important that it doesn't take much to set off a squabble or a war.

Many people in the senior citizen group lived through a depression when parents didn't know what they would even feed their kids because there was no money, no jobs, and no food. Their traditional marriages practiced the idea that men were the hunters and worked outside the home to earn the money the family needed to raise the children and have a comfortable life. Women stayed home managing the business of the home, raised children, and generally deferred to her man to handle the difficult and complex things in life. Many subtle ideas about men and women revolved around this arrangement. For instance, women maintained an air of helplessness and need for protection which supported their feelings of femininity. Her mate was her protector. Money in these families meant power and control and protection and reinforced masculinity. Add to these circumstances the fact that technology had not yet freed women and men from tasks that tied them up for hours so it was physically impossible to do any more than work or take care of the household and family. The division of labor required more clearly assigned roles for marriage partners.

If your sense of masculinity is tied to earning, spending, and saving money, is it any wonder that you will do whatever it takes to control everything about it? And with enhanced feelings of femininity from deferring to your mate to take care of the complicated things in your life like saving and spending money, is it any wonder that you go along with the script?

Our parents dealt with these kinds of issues throughout their marriages. Carolyn's dad, Bob, and Wes (Sr.) played the responsible, masculine role of provider and money manager. They were both good at their role. Laurine and Fran operated their households on whatever allowance their mates deemed adequate. Laurine and Fran also had to learn some pretty fancy maneuvers to buy the things they wanted and needed above and beyond what their mates thought necessary. Their doing so often triggered a war.

Carolyn's dad would say things to her mom like, "why are you so irresponsible about money?" But their script called for her to be the child in relation to money and for Bob to be the responsible father. When that script gets followed it begets father-child interactions. How could Laurine learn to handle money responsibly without ever being responsible for money? Then, add to the mixture, Laurine's desire to reward her hard work and physical and emotional support of her mate and family with some fun and comfort. After all, she had a tough time growing up without any money. Now that she has so much, she wanted to have some fun. But Bob had his sense of what was right and responsible driven by memories of the depression and his idea of masculinity. Saving for a rainy day was the responsible and adult thing to do and every time Laurine spent money he didn't condone she threatened his very idea about himself.

A very similar scenario played itself out in Wes's home. The script both our parents followed reinforced the more submissive, childlike role of our mothers and the more autocratic, fatherly roles of our fathers.

When the roles of marriage partners began to shift, all of these scripts were called into question. First, many of the women in our parents' generation went to work when their mates went to war. For years they performed the work and earned money to take care of the business of the family. When the men came home, they had to leave the work force to give the jobs back to the men. But now they knew how competent and capable they were and didn't want to return to the role of helpless and submissive traditional housewife and mother. Then the cost of living increased. Taxes went up. Technology freed many men and women from the tasks that had tied them up most of the time. And forever challenged were the traditional roles of men and women.

And the shift in roles brought new potential land mines to marriage over money. That's because the money problems stem from the different values people have about money and life. The potential for trouble doesn't go away unless two people have similar beliefs and values about life.

Money problems were the last straw for Carolyn in her first marriage. Neither she, nor her first husband, Steve, were good money managers. The beginning of their marriage followed the more traditional script, but Steve hadn't fully learned his role of traditional provider. Carolyn certainly hadn't learned how to earn or manage money responsibly. She'd witnessed the problems money caused her parents and largely avoided anything to do with managing money. It never occurred to Carolyn that Steve wouldn't handle the money adequately. When their mismanagement of money escalated, neither could salvage any love or passion. Can you envision the scene when Carolyn returned home one day to no money in the bank for food and two IRS agents knocking on their door? Do you have any idea what it's like to have your bank account attached and what you have to go through to get your bank account released? Do you know what it's like to be relegated to bankruptcy to bring some sense of order and responsibility to your life? Do you know what it's like to spend all of your time and energy resolving such problems instead of attending to your family and your life? Do you understand that it took twelve years to untangle the financial mess? Can you imagine the anxiety, fear, insecurity, and anger Carolyn felt? How would they feed their three children? Would Carolyn have to quit school and get a job, undermining her ability to earn a living that really could pay the bills? Would she have to leave school where she was earning straight A's and work for minimum wage? Would she ever be free to mature and take a more responsible role in providing for herself and her children? Carolyn and Steve's mismanagement of money caused many years of debt, insecurity, and fear. Their mismanagement of money and differences about how to earn, spend, and save money, cost them their marriage.

The best thing that happened in the midst of Carolyn's money woes was that she decided she never wanted to live on the edge again and she learned to earn her own money. She learned to set reasonable money goals, based on the way she wanted to live. She figured out what she'd have to do to earn that kind of money, and then she did it.

Another good outcome was that Carolyn's and Steve's children decided early in their lives, that they never wanted to live without enough money themselves. It's a shame that fear and anxiety had to provide their drive to success, but it did, and the outcome has meant work and financial success for them.

But you know what? Carolyn turned around and chose the wrong partner again, just because he was stable and passive and never kept secrets. He was so stable and passive that he had no self. She traded financial security for a partner whose views of life were so different on other important issues that she ended up in a marriage of convenience. It didn't take her long to yearn for a partner with more of an adventuresome spirit engaged in the challenges of life. She learned that of the differences that make a difference, none were more important than the other was. Differences that make a difference are all important.

A new scenario plagues Maggie and Jake. Maggie came to therapy at the age of 25. She felt unhappy in her marriage and didn't know if she should stay or leave. Maggie, being the youngest of several children, had learned to take good care of herself. She'd always felt responsible for earning her own paycheck and for appropriate money management. She went to college, earned a degree in early childhood education, and got a job. During her college years she worked, paid her own school bills, and saved several thousand dollars. She inherited some money from a relative. By the time Maggie married Jake, she'd accumulated a decent sum of money of her own.

As is often the case, Maggie married someone very different from her in many ways. Jake came from a family with plenty of money and had never had to fend for himself. Jake's more impulsive nature led him to do risky things in many ways. Money issues in their marriage may end it.

Jake wants Maggie to consent to spend her money any way he sees fit. Maggie disagrees and is enraged that Jake believes he has the right to tell her how to use her money. The way Jake spends money makes Maggie anxious and insecure. She says, "why does he think he has the right to tell me what to do with my own money? I just don't want to spend it the way he says I should."

Jake's impulsive behavior fuels Maggie's distrust and insecurity. Maggie's distrust and insecurity fuels Jake's sense that Maggie is disloyal and selfish. After two and a half years of marriage, they have separate bank accounts, Maggie is learning not to tell Jake anything about her money; they pay bills separately with his money and her money. The money they got for their wedding is the only money that Maggie agrees belongs to them both equally. But that means to Maggie that she gets an equal say in how it gets managed. Jake thinks it means he should guide their decisions about how to spend it and Maggie should defer to him.

We hope you noticed that Maggie's and Jake's money trouble comes from differences in the way they believe money should be earned, spent, and saved, and from differences in their expectations of marriage and their roles in the marriage.

The ending of this story is that only time will tell if Jake's views on money are a function of his inexperience in life and immaturity. If it is, he may change as he gains maturity. However, if Jake's views about money represent deeper values about life, it's very likely his views will never change. Nor should they have to. But if they don't, Maggie and Jake will either have a bad marriage, dueling over money for years, or they'll have a marriage of convenience with no real passion, because they'll find a way to peacefully coexist with separate money, or they'll divorce. They'll never have the possibility of a great marriage.

Money problems are never simple. They get tangled with many other issues so working them out takes skill and a lot of hard work. Can you see how having different ideas about earning, spending, and saving money can have an enormous impact on marriage? Do you want it to cause trouble in your marriage? Money problems can be kept to a minimum by marrying someone with ideas about money that are similar to your own.

Problems with Sexual Intimacy

One of the most wonderful gifts of marriage to the right partner is sexual intimacy. The unity, love, joy, and physical feelings of well-being (peace) of a spiritual connection with a higher power is all that can top the unity, love, joy, and peace generated from satisfying sexual intimacy. It's possible that, as spiritual beings in human form, satisfying sexual intimacy is designed to remind us of the unity, love, joy, and peace of a higher power.

Having sex is relatively easy. Having satisfying sexual intimacy requires mutual trust, admiration, respect, emotional and physical safety, similar sexual drives and interests, good mental and physical health, strong and fit bodies, privacy, and knowledge about male and female sexual response. Either kind of sex can beget children. Children as a possible result of sex elevate sex to a high level of need for responsibility. The possibility of sterility, illness, and death from irresponsible sex requires forethought and the decision to have sex rather than just having sex when the desire strikes. The potential for a great marriage when satisfying sexual intimacy exists requires that sex be held in highest esteem.

One of the reasons we get married is to have responsible sex.

Sex is a powerful tool with which to fortify or destroy a marriage. Sex deepens the intimacy and bond between two people. Having a sexual relationship with a new partner before you know how well you match on the differences that make a difference can attach you to the wrong partner, causing pain and heartache when the incompatibility is finally realized. Both alternatives in having to decide whether to stay in a marriage with no potential for satisfying happiness or to leave are equally painful and destructive.

When something related to sex goes wrong in a marriage, few things can be more miserable and destructive. If you're not getting enough sex, you feel physically and emotionally deprived. If your partner wants more sex than you want, you feel pressured. If sex is dissatisfying, you distract yourself with other activities and grow apart or you yearn for satisfaction. Because sex is a need, not just a want, a poor sexual relationship in your marriage can cause you to look outside of your marriage for sexual satisfaction. If you don't get enough support and respect from your partner, sex can be used to find support and respect outside your marriage.

Do you want to spend your adult life yearning for sexual intimacy and satisfaction? Do you want your partner to yearn for sexual intimacy and satisfaction? Do you want to be faced with the dilemma of adultery or chronic dissatisfaction of a basic need for either you or your partner? Do you want to be responsible for depriving your mate or yourself of the pleasure, emotional support, validation, and comfort of sexual intimacy? Do you want to deprive your partner or yourself of physical health?

When marriage partners have problems with sexual intimacy few things can feel worse.

Susan, a 68 year old woman, came to therapy because her husband had recently begun to experience impotence. Fred is 72, and until now, has never had difficulty with his sexual performance. In exploring the circumstances surrounding the impotence Carolyn and her patient uncovered several other marital problems, all of which could be related some how to the sexual problem this couple now has.

Primary was Susan's vaginal dryness, which caused painful intercourse. Susan had begun to avoid sexual intimacy because of the pain that intercourse caused. She'd tolerated painful intercourse for quite a while, just as she'd tolerated no orgasms for herself as a result of her sexual experiences with Fred for forty years. Her tolerance without complaint actually deepened their problem and had prevented any kind of intimacy over the course of their marriage. Like so many others, Susan was afraid to hurt her husband's feelings by telling him he wasn't satisfying her. She also believed the myth that women just weren't supposed to like sex as much as men. She felt she should protect her husband's ego. Susan believed in self-sacrifice.

The chronic feelings of resentment over dissatisfying sex caused Susan to grow further apart from her husband. Fred busied himself with work, also believing the myth that women don't like sex as much as men. Occasionally, he felt angry and puzzled at Susan's emotional distance and, at times, her irritability and hostility. Since Susan had never told him of her dissatisfaction, Fred never learned anything other than minimal foreplay and intercourse, satisfying himself and believing that Susan must be satisfied too. Lack of knowledge seriously limited their sexual repertoire. Neither had any idea what to do about Fred's impotence. They lacked the capacity for intimacy that such a problem requires in order to find a solution. Even with new information, Susan and Fred could not overcome their inhibitions after a 40-year marriage that lacked intimacy. They didn't divorce, but they will finish their days in a marriage that lacks unity, joy, peace, and love. Can you imagine anything lonelier than this marriage?

Outside Pressures from Work, Family and Friends

How many of you know someone who feels as

though they are in a competition with someone or something just to win a few minutes with their mate? How many of you know someone who must fight for his or her mate to defend them when questioned or challenged by their mate's mother or father? How many of you know someone who carries out traditions of their family of origin in their new marriage just as they did as a child so they won't be disowned? How many of you have seen someone you love alone most of the time, because their mate spends most of his or her time at work or with his or her family of origin or other friends?

Sure you can distract yourself for a while. You can get a life of your own to make up for no time together as mates. You can even talk yourself into believing that your parents raised you, they deserve your total allegiance. Neither will give you a great marriage. Both contribute to a poor marriage or a marriage of convenience.

Marriage forms a new family unit and its first task is to shift your primary loyalty and allegiance to the new family unit. What that means is that the new bride and groom are responsible to protect the boundaries they've formed together by their union. You must shift your primary loyalty from your family of origin, your parents, to your mate. You must blend the customs and traditions and ways of daily life of both mates, finding your own expression of what you believe and stand for. You must establish your own priorities and time tables.

Here is one more place where similarities in basic values will provide the solid foundation for the formation of a new family relatively easily. When your values are similar, you have much less work to do to blend the styles of each of your families of origin. You have a much greater ability to satisfy your parents with your own style, because the blend will comprise itself of behaviors, beliefs, and attitudes that both families understand. The separation from the family of origin to the new family won't feel nearly as threatening as it would for families that differ widely on certain values.

When you have a constant bombardment on the new marriage of outside influences, that stresses the new couple to their limit. It matters little where the bombardment originates. Whether it is work or relatives or friends, having to choose loyalties stresses everyone. Defending your mate and your time together must happen. That defense takes time and energy. Obviously, the less time and energy you must spend on insisting that your marriage deserves first place, the more time and energy you'll have for life's challenges.

Bonnie and Walt initially admired each other for similar ambition and their desired lifestyle. Both took pride in Walt's work accomplishments. Bonnie's willing sacrifice of time together with Walt allowed Walt to choose work over their time together. They got the house they wanted. They kept up with the Jones's. But while Walt is off working and feeling good about what he does, Bonnie's had to find a life of her own. She does okay and stays very busy. But they have a very sad and lonely marriage. Unfortunately, since the approval of others and outshining others is their way of feeling good about themselves it leaves little room for thinking for themselves and forging a marriage together. They're together, but in a marriage that is barely functional.

Being together in a house, having children together, having bank accounts together are the business of marriage, but being together, having fun together, having great sex, being fully engaged and interested in each others lives, is marriage.

Bonnie and Walt illustrate that while you need to have similar values on the differences that make a difference, you also have to have those values based on thinking for yourself – the values must be yours and not belong to someone else. To learn to think for yourself you must outgrow your need for approval solely from others. Not learning to think for yourself is the easy way out, it pleases certain people that value obedience, and it keeps you mired in childhood's need for survival based on dependence. In Bonnie and Walt's case, it means looking good and feeling lousy.

Sara and Rick have been married ten years. When they married, Rick had never been married and had lived at home. He was 38 when they married. Most of the spare time Rick has, other than work gets spent helping his mother around her house. How do you think Sara feels that her husband spends his time and energy on his mother rather than on her and their family? Do you think she feels she means as much or more to him than his mother? Do you think Sara should be left to her own devices to run their home, while Rick runs his mother's home? Oh yes, Rick's dad is alive and well, living in the same house as Rick's mother.

Twenty-two years into their marriage, Wes (Sr.) neglected to support his wife at a family get-together. Wes and Fran were visiting Wes's parents along with their four children. Wes's sister had just learned to make a certain kind of cake. She was thirteen and taking pride in the homemaking skills her mother was teaching her. At the table, Wes's sister made a comment about how she likes her cake better than the one they were eating, which Wes's (Sr.) mother had made. The grandmother started scolding her granddaughter for being rude and said that Fran was a terrible mother, teaching her children to be ungrateful. Wes Senior's Mother began to cry so he put his arms around his mother and scolded his wife for causing trouble. Taking her granddaughter's comment personally was bad enough, but then the grandmother proceeded to compete with her son's wife. And, 22 years into the marriage, Wes Sr. defended his mother and lets Fran fend for herself. Can you imagine how Fran felt being abandoned by her mate like that? Can you imagine how much that hurt Fran? The emotional pain of that incident lingers thirty years later.

Connie and Joe have a constant battle going over how to raise the children and the neatness of their house. Joe believes the way he grew up was the best and only way to do things. Today, when his mother or sisters suggest something should be a certain way, Joe defends them. Connie isn't neat enough. Connie doesn't handle the kids right. Joe has never learned that many right ways exist to do things. Joe hasn't learned that he is no longer a child that needs to win the approval of his mother and sisters to survive. That's because while he was growing up his mother made it clear that, unless Joe did as she said, she would withdraw her love. His need to win his mother's approval supercedes his need to be supportive and validating to his wife. His inability to blend his style with Connie's style, finding the best style suitable to their life and family, limits their marriage to mediocre at best. Fortunately, they have some positive aspects to their marriage so they have avoided divorce, but at times their marriage borders on emotional and verbal abuse. They suffer much emotional pain over the issues raised about where Joe's loyalty belongs.

Many variations on this theme abound. We're sure you can identify these kinds of problems if you take a look around you. Do you want your marriage to be limited by the drain of outside influences on your life?

Marital Land Mines Cause Misery and Divorce

You need to understand that these problems are pervasive in our marriages and cause misery and divorce. All of the predominant issues relate to differences that make a difference. To date, the best most therapists and marriage counselors can come up with to contend with these pervasive problems is to help you improve your relationship skills to make the differences less destructive. Unfortunately, even with brilliantly polished relationship skills, if you end up with a marriage partner that has important differences from you, you won't achieve a great marriage. You'll spend your time and energy on endless negotiation and compromise and talking yourself into accepting disappointment, and not having what you want.

Spending your life in a marriage to the wrong partner is a sure way to a short leash on life. Pun intended. Something far better exists. Contrary to popular belief, marriage doesn't have to be difficult. You don't have to be afraid of marriage because so many crash and burn. Don't let cynicism stop you from what you really want. Just don't make the same mistakes they make. Find the right marriage partner.

We're going to show you how.

3

Challenge the Myth!

You Can Have a Great Marriage With Your Perfect Partner

The saddest part of poor marriages and marriages of convenience is that it doesn't have to be that way.

Unleash yourself.

Other than knowing yourself and acting with integrity, nothing is more important in this human life than choosing the right marriage partner. Your marriage will affect your life in profound ways, for better or for worse. Your marriage will influence your life and the lives of those around you for generations to come.

Accept the challenge. Refuse to accept that marriage is hard work to the inevitable never perfect partner.

If you haven't reached a level of self-esteem that assures that you deserve a great marriage, then do it for your children. Break the cycle of poor role models.

Offer yourself the opportunity to be the best you can be.

Here are the simple truths about creating a great marriage.

Of What are Great Marriages Made?

Great marriages are made of:

-A high level of compatibility on each of the 16 differences that make a difference which offers a natural acceptance, respect, and approval to each
-Two adults with good relationship skills that reflect a mutual and reciprocal respect, competence in handling daily living, the ability to set reasonable goals and accomplish them, an active interest in each other's lives, and the ability to cope constructively with crises and maintain a spirit of personal growth
-Great sex

Do You Know What a Great Marriage Can Give You?

Once you realize what a great marriage offers, you'll be hard pressed to have anything less.

A great marriage:

- -Prevents all of the land mines described to you in Chapter 2
- -Liberates time and energy for life's tasks, and provides a platform from which to meet other challenges your life brings
- -Offers you the chance to be the best you can be at work, play, and relationships
- -Contributes to physical and mental health
- -Balances the work of life with fun and recreation
- -Gives you more energy
- -Contributes to a variety of successes in work and play
- -Provides an opportunity for your children to see healthy role models for marriage and life so they can become the best they can be
- -Contributes to the health of your community

Our Definition of a Great Marriage

A great marriage is a marriage of two healthy adults that manage life competently. Each partner offers the other acceptance and the emotional safety to be who he or she naturally is. Differences of opinions are a minor part of their life and handled with mutual respect. Conflict is a small part of their life and is managed respectfully, in a friendly and supportive manner. In a great marriage both partners win all of the time.

Partners in a great marriage handle the tasks of daily living smoothly and easily. Partners in a great marriage know how to set healthy limits for their children and provide the best possible environment for children to learn how to select the right marriage partner and how to have a great marriage.

A great marriage is fun. A great marriage works all of its own accord. Gone forever is the need to work hard to make it work.

Intimacy

A great marriage has a high level of intimacy. Intimacy is the act of disclosing your deepest joys and fears, your real thoughts and feelings to another person. Intimacy is the quality of a relationship that prevents our feeling alone in the world and facilitates emotional support and validation for each partner. Intimacy contributes to the prevention of heart disease and other physical illness. (Read James Lynch's book, The Broken Heart.)

Partners in a great marriage are not afraid of intimacy. They seek intimacy and they want to provide emotional safety for intimacy for their partner.

Acceptance vs. Tolerance

Do you know the difference? Acceptance is rooted in a natural respect and admiration for similar values. Tolerance means sufferance or open-mindedness. Acceptance lets you keep your own values, tolerance means you will tolerate someone else's values at the expense of your values. With acceptance both partners win. With tolerance one partner loses. Acceptance allows the maintenance of your integrity. Tolerance prevents integrity.

Would you rather find acceptance or tolerance in your marriage?

Tolerance is what happens in marriages to the wrong partner. Acceptance is easy when married to your perfect partner.

Emotional Safety

Emotional safety means offering respect. Equal weight is given each partner's need to win and be understood. When your partner receives the disclosures you make, they don't ridicule, call you names, shame, or humiliate.

The climate of a great marriage offers emotional safety.

Great Sex

How would you like to have great sex? In a survey we conducted, we learned that sex is important to both men and women. In fact, more women than men said sex was very important. That surprised many people because they'd been told, repeatedly, that women just don't like sex, especially not as much as men.

Sexual intimacy is an important part of intimacy. In a great marriage, sex offers a personal expression of affection, admiration, and appreciation. Both partners' need for sexual satisfaction is met in a great marriage.

Great sex includes physical and emotional satisfaction. Great sex contributes to physical and emotional health. Great sex fortifies your marital bond and attachment.

Great sex involves two partners that have similar sex drives and like similar demonstrations of affection. Emotional safety and acceptance provide for unguarded performance and communication of desires. Partners seek to learn what satisfies their partner and provide it for them. Partners know about the basics of male and female sexual response and anatomy. Robust physical health, fitness, and good nutrition fuel great sex.

Great sex with perfect partners grows better with time.

Great sex is so important that we're going to give you our personal example of great sex to make up for any knowledge deficit you may have. You'll find our example in Chapter 9.

Our Experience with Perfect Partners

It took both of us much time and heartache before we figured out how to improve our choices and chances of finding the right partner. The difference between marriage to the wrong partner and marriage to the right partner is the difference between a bad marriage and a great marriage. What a difference, when you marry the right person. We find ourselves repeating that comment over and over: what a difference!

Carolyn never gave up hope that she'd find the perfect partner and have a great marriage. But her son, Ryan, and daughter-in-law, Amanda and their marriage inspired her to know it was possible. Not having seen other great marriages, Carolyn had hoped for one, but doubt lurked in the shadows of her thinking. That is, until she saw the difference in their relationship.

Watching Ryan and Amanda together is like a breath of fresh air. Being with them is energizing. Friendly, respectful, helpful, loving, supportive, nurturing, and playful are all adjectives that describe their interactions with each other. Until Carolyn met Wes she had never seen a happier couple. Their happiness and optimism affects everyone with whom they come in contact. Conflict and disagreements are minor and handled respectfully, so both win. And they never last long. One time, after Carolyn's oldest son, Jeff, had suffered a heartbreaking split with someone he thought he should marry, Jeff said to Carolyn, "how'd Ryan do it so well? How'd he know how to find the right person?"

Their interactions with each other aren't the only thing positive in their lives. Their careers have flourished. We've watched them set goals, individually and as a couple, and we haven't seen them miss achieving one of them yet. They finished undergraduate degrees. They both worked at jobs directly related to what they wanted to do to gain experience. They wanted to return to graduate school. And they wanted to go as close to the top as they could manage. They managed quitting their jobs and graduate school easily and smoothly, mutually supportive of each other. Ryan got his MBA from a top school and Amanda recently graduated from law school and passed her bar exam.

They've both gotten top-paying jobs in the exact place they want to live. They're in the process of buying a house exactly where they want to live.

You may be tempted to say they must be special. Or they must have all the luck. Of course they're special, but neither attained these goals magically.

Amanda had to help put herself through college. She's still paying off undergraduate loans. She'll soon be paying off the loans she needed to go to law school. She worked as a residential assistant in her dorm to help pay for her expenses.

It isn't luck or privilege that fulfilled Amanda's dreams. It was determination and the expectation that she could do anything she really wanted to do.

Ryan didn't have the attainment of his goals handed to him either. He worked from the age of 14. He helped put himself through his undergraduate degree at a state university. He never worked less than 30 hours a week during college. He graduated with a 2.8 and worried that he wouldn't be able to get into graduate school. But the fact that he'd worked so hard to finish and that he'd bought a house (as a college student and rented the rooms to pay the mortgage to other college students) scraping together every cent he could, impressed prospective employers and graduate school admissions officers. He got the job he wanted and was accepted to all of the graduate schools to which he applied except the number one school in the country. When Ryan found out he hadn't been accepted to the number one school, he said, "it's nice to have a realistic estimation of my limits."

And, most important of all, they found each other. Their relationship and marriage are the result of personal characteristics that help them live effectively. Their marriage has made the attainment of all of their other goals easier. Their marriage energizes them.

Once Carolyn experienced the success of her son's marriage, she knew she wanted that for herself. She began to examine the elements of their relationship in comparison to what hadn't worked for her in the past and with all of the troubled relationships of patients she's treated. Little-by-little, the picture came together.

When Carolyn found Wes and felt the difference herself, she knew she had to try and help others have it too.

Meanwhile, Wes was looking for his own perfect partner. Even though the break up of his marriage was a big disappointment, the idea that he could find someone that would fall in love with him filled him with hope.

Looking for a new marriage partner wasn't easy, but Wes took the plunge and decided to go about looking in as effective a way as possible. It wasn't until after they found each other, that Wes closely examined how they'd done it, so the process he went through didn't have the benefit of knowing how.

Having been interested in efficiency and effectiveness most of his work career, he one day noticed the book, The 7 Habits of Highly Effective People, by Stephen Covey, in a coworker's hand. He looked it over and bought one for himself. It didn't take Wes long to realize that everything Covey had to say about effectiveness also applied to finding the right marriage partner. He looked for ways to apply the ideas in his search.

And Wes knew what he didn't want. He had a good idea of what doesn't work. He looked for emotional safety to re-build his self-confidence.

Once finding each other, Carolyn knew that she was looking at the second great marriage she'd ever seen. We marvel at the difference our relationship makes in our lives.

The same friendly, safe, helpful, respectful, loving, nurturing, supportive, playful interactions between Ryan and Amanda mark our marriage.

Sex is important to both of us, and we've never been so sexually satisfied. We're affectionate in the same ways. We're six weeks apart in age, so our backgrounds are similar in regard to the music, arts, and politics of our generation. Our ambitions and educational levels are similar. We like casual living and agree on where we want to live. Our children are nearly all on their own. We look forward to traveling and an early retirement. Our leisure interests are the same. We love to go to good restaurants and like the same movies. We like to work out together. We eat similar food with an eye on good nutrition and fitness. We like to ride our bikes and go for walks. Our religious and spiritual backgrounds are identical and we have the same level of interest and practice of our beliefs. We agree on how much money we want to make and how we want to make it. We agree on how to save, invest, and spend money. Marriage is important to both of us and we both value loving each other. Our relationship is at the top of our priorities. We're each other's best friends. We'd rather do things with each other than anyone else. We can tell each other our deepest joys and fears. We can think out loud and know we're safe from ridicule and shame. We can't imagine having a better partner. We can count on each other and lean temporarily when the going gets tough and when we need that extra push. We can count on each other to handle life competently. We can count on each other to live with honesty and integrity. We can count on each other to achieve success in our personal and work lives.

Sure, we have some differences, but they're differences that don't make much difference. The differences don't ask us to compromise our values; they don't ask that we deny ourselves our integrity. We're not clones. We're anything but bored. Having so much safety, security, and energy from our relationship evokes tremendous curiosity for new experiences and new learning. Having similar values is not the same as loving only a reproduction of us. Our similarities are not an exercise in narcissistic love.

Our marriage is exhilarating. Our relationship is free of the constant negotiation and compromise that plagues most marriages. Our disagreements are few, our conflict minimal.

The emotional safety and acceptance that comes to us naturally, liberates us to conquer new challenges.

Our relationship makes a remarkable difference in our lives. We're doing the work we want to do. We're physically and mentally healthier. We take better care of ourselves. We seek interesting challenges. We're refocusing our energy on helping as many people as we can have their own great marriage by finding their perfect partner. We have a lot more fun.

The hope and success replacing the despair of Carolyn's patients who've tried our methods is deeply inspiring. One patient recently told Carolyn, "I come in here full of despair and I always leave full of hope". Another patient jumped for joy when she learned that a young man she was going to meet was schooled in our ideas and knew about the 16 differences that make a difference and great marriages.

Carolyn's youngest son, Todd, and his new wife Alysa have joined the ranks of great marriages. And, yes, Jeff found his own perfect partner too.

With deepest joy and love, we report that:

-Men are not all the same
-Women are not all the same
-And, not all marriages take a lot of hard
 work

No One Says Finding the Right Partner is Easy, But it Doesn't Have to Be Hard Either

You're either going to work now to find the right partner or you're going to work later, endlessly trying to survive marriage to the wrong partner.

Ask yourself: Has whatever you've been doing to find a marriage partner worked? Have you seen what others do to find a marriage partner result in a great marriage? Since you're reading this book, we doubt it.

Wouldn't you rather put your time and energy in up front, and find your perfect partner, than spend the rest of your life working hard to make it work? Wouldn't your rather get it right before all the anguish and pain of marriage to the wrong partner and then divorce?

Investing your time and energy up front to find the right partner takes work. Most things worth having do take some effort, but maybe not as much as you think. Especially when you know what to do.

Now that you know what a great marriage is all about and you've seen the rewards, we're confident you'll be happy to put your work in up front. We've drawn a detailed map for you to follow, making your work to find the right partner less difficult. And the things you do to find the right partner for marriage are also the things you do to help you manage your life constructively in every other area. Your investment will provide infinite returns.

Come with us and we'll show you how.

You don't have to marry:
Only for physical attraction

Instead, you can:
Make certain you match on the 16 differences that make a difference and make certain the other person is ready for marriage by asking yourself five crucial questions

You don't have to marry:
Because they seem familiar

Instead, you can:
Make sure you've finished unfinished business from your past, freeing yourself to choose in the here and now, on purpose, and in your own best interest

You don't have to marry:
Because your choices are limited

Instead, you can:
Dramatically enlarge your pool of choices

You don't have to marry:
Someone because they like you based on an act

designed to gain approval

Instead, you can:
Know who you really are, match your behavior to the real you, and like yourself

You don't have to marry:
Someone that can do the things you can't do

Instead, you can:
Become competent at tasks of daily living yourself and learn how to turn to appropriate resources to do the things at which you aren't skillful

You don't have to marry:
Because this prince or princess can give you things you've dreamed of having

Instead, you can:
Find a real person that has similar life views and values and together you can achieve your goals

You don't have to marry:
To win the approval of others

Instead, you can:
Think for yourself, find your perfect partner, and win your own approval

You don't have to marry:
The wrong person because you don't know yourself

Instead, you can:
Spend some time getting to know yourself and what you want

You don't have to marry:
Because you believe you're at the mercy of falling in love

Instead, you can:
Choose when to fall in love

You don't have to marry:
Someone that seems good enough, believing mismatches are natural

Instead, you can:
Find your perfect partner

Part II

You Can Find Your Perfect Partner if You Know Who You Are and What You Want

4

Get Your Head Straight

The First Step to Finding Your Perfect Partner

Develop a wonderful relationship with yourself. Getting your head straight is hard, so what are the benefits? Getting your head straight :

- -helps you grow up – marriage is for adults
- -helps you avoid having to change your partner
- -is more satifying work than struggling to make marriage to the wrong partner work
- -helps you trust yourself so you can trust others if they're worthy of trust
- -helps you to believe in yourself which is attractive to others

-helps you to feel attracted to competent
partners who match you well on 16
specific characteristics
-increases your ability to withstand
rejection and competition
-helps you know what you want from your
partner and marriage
-enables you to avoid the reasons people
marry the wrong person
-enables you to accomplish nine marital
tasks
-dramatically increases your chances for
a great marriage to the perfect partner
-dramatically increases your chances for
great sex

The way you feel about yourself influences how
you relate to every person and situation in your
life. The way you feel about yourself affects how
you think about and interpret events. The way
you understand what is happening in your life
filters through the way you feel about yourself.
When you feel good about yourself, you convey
to others that you believe in yourself. When you
feel good about yourself, getting others to
believe in you is relatively easy. When you feel
good about yourself, you expect that good will
happen to you. Your expectation of happy endings results in happy endings.

Carolyn worked on herself to understand
the choices she made. She diligently examined
her experiences, behaviors, and their results.
Her early relationships were remarkable in that
she consistently chose dominating men. Since

Carolyn didn't feel competent and adequate on her own, she found herself attracted to men who liked to run the show. And those men were attracted to her because she submitted to their demands.

With determination and over time, Carolyn grew up. She decided she needed to take care of herself, to stop depending on others to make life work right. For one thing, life wasn't working right at all with the men that she selected in control. Carolyn decided to take responsibility for her life.

As she learned the skills necessary to be competent and effective, her life changed decidedly for the better. As Carolyn matured, the feelings she had about herself changed. Maturation gave birth to an inner strength and knowing that helped her in every aspect of her life. From that moment on, every step she took came from a sense of adequacy. Growing up resulted in finding the perfect partner and a great marriage, something she never gave up hope of finding.

Getting Your Head Straight Means Knowing The Real You

What's your favorite food? What's your favorite color? Where would you like to live? In what kind of house? With what kind of furniture? What kind of job do you want? Do you want to get married? Do you want to have children? What do you believe in? How do you think a wife or husband is supposed to act? What do you think is good parenting? What kind of car do you want to drive? Do you like movies? What kind of movies? What's your favorite music? Do you like air conditioning? Do you like to sleep with the windows open? How do you act when you're angry? When you're hurt? When you're happy?

One primary task of this human life is to become who you truly are. A hallmark of maturity is the ability to think for yourself. You must not blindly accept all that you've heard from others, but you must challenge ideas and learn about life from your own experience. You must live your values – not someone else's values. You must go to the trouble of having your own values and living by them.

Before you move on to defining who your perfect partner is, you must know yourself well. Use the following list to be very specific about who you are. Describe yourself. Remember, we're asking about your values – beliefs and practices that would compromise your integrity if you were to negotiate and compromise. For an equal partnership and to avoid power struggles you must resist asking yourself or your partner to compromise your values and integrity. Some things are non-negotiable.

We recommend keeping a written log of your answers to these questions about yourself. A journal will do fine. A log on the computer for those of you that prefer the computer would be another excellent means of keeping written records of your thoughts as you progress in this process.

The act of writing will help your sub-con-

scious mind use the information to your benefit. If you'd like more intensive help and structure, our workbooks, Find Your Perfect Partner
Step-By-Step and When You Think You've
Found Your Perfect Partner Step-By-Step have
several exercises that can help you get your
head straight and know what you want. See the
back of this book to order or find them in your
local bookstore.

16 Things You Need To Know About Yourself

Sex drives/sexual interests/demonstration of affection – how often do you like to have sex?
How important is sex to you? How do you
express your sexuality? Do you like to hold
hands? How adventuresome are your sexual
interests? What do you think and practice
about birth control issues?

Age – What is your age? What kinds of beliefs
and practices do you have because of the times
in which you've grown up? The closer you are in
age, the closer interests of your era will be. Age
is related to many of the other characteristics.

Health and fitness, including the habits of smoking, drinking, or using drugs – What are
your beliefs and practices in regard to health
and fitness? Do you exercise regularly? What
kind of diet and eating pattern do you follow?
What habits do you have or don't you like that

would affect how you feel about your marriage partner? What are your beliefs and practices about smoking, drinking, and using drugs? How will your beliefs and practices affect your marriage and family life?

Where to live – Where do you want to live? Will your career dictate where to live? Where do you want to live in regard to your extended family? How does your health impact on where you want to live? Do you have any allergies that would impact where you live? What about climate?

Education/Intelligence – What do you like to talk about? How do you problem solve? What are your educational and intellectual ambitions? How will getting your education affect your marriage and family life?

Lifestyle (Formal versus Informal) – Do you like to take off your shoes and put your feet up? Do you like everything in its place or is your home some place to let your hair down? Would you rather entertain at a backyard barbecue or a dinner party? Are you child and family oriented or career and philanthropically oriented?

Views about work/Level of ambition – What are your ambitions about work and career? How do you balance work and pleasure? What kind of hours will you work? How will your work impact marriage and family life?

Views on how to handle and spend money –

How do you want to spend, save and invest? What are your short and long-term financial goals? What meanings do you attach to money? Was money an issue in your family of origin? Do you know how to manage money? How should money be managed in a marriage?

Expectations of marriage/relationship – How much time do you want to spend with your spouse? Do you want to be best friends or share confidences with other best friends, too? What are your expectations of marriage? What do you believe about roles of men and women in marriage?

Physical characteristics attractive to you – What about looks are important to you? What kinds of physical characteristics turn you on?

Religious beliefs and practices – What are your religious beliefs and practices? To what extent can you blend your beliefs and practices with your spouse? How will your beliefs and practices affect your marriage and family life? Does religion play a major or minor role in your life? How do you want to raise your children in regard to religion? Have you thought about the difference between spirituality and organized religion? What do you believe about spirituality and organized religion?

Political beliefs and practices – What are your beliefs and practices in regard to politics? Do politics play a major or minor role in your life? What role do you anticipate politics will play in your future? How do political beliefs relate to psychology and the way people behave? Have you thought about your political beliefs separate from your parents' political beliefs?

Children: Having them and raising them – Do you want children? When and how many? How will you raise your children? What roles do each parent play? How will you discipline? What's your parenting style? Have you had much experience with children? Do you need more experience with children in order to know more about your style with them? What kinds of issues from your childhood home might affect the way you raise your children and the expectations you have of your partner's parenting?

Life stage – when do you want to get married? When will you be ready to have children? Will you be working on your career and raising a family at the same time? What is the timing of your financial goals? When do you intend to retire? What life tasks will you be engaged in and when? How do you want to time events in your life?

Common leisure interests – What do you like to do in your leisure time? How do you balance fun and work? How much time do you want to spend on leisure activities?

Energy levels – How much energy do you have to work and play? What time of the day are you the most energetic? The least energetic? Is your energy introverted or extraverted – do you spend your energy on mental and intellectual pursuits or physically?

Wes grew up feeling relatively safe and secure accepting the world as his parents portrayed it. His parents' lives seemed to run smoothly, the children grew up with few problems, and life was good. But as Wes has recently become aware, the choices he made in his career and a marriage partner fit his parents' pattern not his own needs. Wes felt chronic disappointment and dissatisfaction with his life.

Wes and his first wife limped along in their marriage, neither satisfied nor happy. Wes limped along in his work. After eighteen years, his marriage fell apart.

For the first time, Wes had to take care of himself. He learned to manage the tasks of daily living on his own. He too, began to study and examine his life and his choices and their results. Without the distractions of meeting everyone else's needs, slowly he got to know himself, his needs, and what he wanted from life. He got to know the real Wes. Realizing that innovation and creativity excite him enough to challenge the status quo, Wes started making choices based on who he really was. His life blossomed into a great marriage, great sex, and the risk and exhilaration of working for himself.

Not knowing the real you can also be a problem when you have an over-inflated view of yourself, as is the case with Debbie. Debbie grew up believing she could do no wrong. Others in Debbie's life smoothed over events and interactions so Debbie never got an accurate picture of what she could and couldn't do. Leaving home gave Debbie a real run for her money because most people outside of Debbie's family had a more realistic estimation about what Debbie could and couldn't do. If certain relatives showed the slightest interest in her life, she interpreted the interest as an attempt to control her. Her college professors incurred her wrath by their mere criticism of her work. Boyfriends were either totally out of step with her educationally, never having graduated from high school let alone attended college, or non-existent because no one adores Debbie at the level to which she's accustomed. Having never considered others' opinions and suggestions, she's so insensitive to others' ideas that she usually can't hear anything helpful. In Debbie's case, her inflated sense of self is holding her back from considerable achievement and happiness.

Honest answers to the questions above, and others like them, tell you who you are. But it isn't enough to know the real you; you have to act like the real you, too.

Getting Your Head Straight Means Being Yourself

Being yourself means matching your actions to the real you. Being yourself is behaving in a manner that supports your beliefs. Being you is what integrity is all about.

Suzanne didn't love Rusty, but she

thought he'd make a good provider and father. During two years of dating, living together, and then the early years of their marriage, Suzanne resisted asserting herself in her marriage. She accommodated to Rusty's needs day after day. Over time she stored up layer upon layer of resentment, anger, and disappointment. Finally, one day she could contain herself no more and the real Suzanne came spilling forth.

Rusty had no idea Suzanne's resentment was building. He thought everyone was happy, even if life was nothing spectacular.

Suzanne's eruption of emotion changed their lives forever, ending a loveless marriage. By then, Suzanne had become hardened about men, blamed Rusty for being bad instead of different, and believed he should change for her; Rusty felt betrayed and humiliated, and two children had been deprived of role models that would teach them about healthy adult male and female behavior and relationships.

If the real you includes feeling angry when someone puts you down, what do you do about it? Do you pretend like you're okay, or do you set limits on the other person's hostile remarks? If you don't want to do something someone's asked you to do, do you do what he or she wants, or do you say, "no?" If you believe in taking good care of yourself, do you follow a routine of good nutrition and exercise, rest and recreation balanced with satisfying work? Or do you just tell others they should follow a routine of good nutrition and exercise, rest and recreation balanced with satisfying work, without taking good care of yourself? Do you practice what you preach?

How can you know what you want if you don't know your likes and dislikes? If you've imitated your parents' likes and dislikes, without thinking about what they say and do, are you sure they fit you and your life? If you act without thinking, how can you take control of your life? If you adopt others' values without thinking about what seems right to you, how can you be sure those values apply to your life today? What good is the real you if nobody knows the real you? How can you match with your perfect partner if the real you is hidden?

And it isn't good enough to know the real you and to act like the real you, unless you like the real you.

Getting Your Head Straight Means Liking Yourself

If there's something about the real you that you don't like, how are you going to convince another person to like the real you? If you can't like yourself, how will you ever believe another person could like the real you?

Liking yourself has a lot to do with whether your behavior matches who you really are. Liking yourself means you're living up to your own expectations. Realistic expectations that are high enough to stretch you a bit, that is. Living up to expectations that have been lowered to meet someone else's standards, or some preconceived notion of yourself (your lazy, you'll never amount to anything, your stupid...) doesn't achieve liking yourself. Only competence and maintaining your integrity gives you good feelings about yourself.

Don't confuse acceptance with liking. Acceptance means you're willing to see the reality of what's going on whether you like it or not. Acceptance doesn't necessarily mean you like what's going on.

What kind of a reputation do you have with yourself? How do you treat your beliefs? Do you make reasonable promises? Do you keep your promises? How would you describe the perfect person? Is your description realistic; is that description humanly possible? How close does your description of the perfect person come to the real you? Do you trust yourself? Do you believe what you see and hear? Do you believe you can handle most of life's tasks? How do you talk to yourself? Do you feel better or worse about yourself because of what you say to yourself? Can you count on yourself to find solutions to problems?

Sarah's laid back, relaxed style of approaching life had been labeled laziness throughout her childhood. Unfortunately, at twenty-nine, Sarah believed she was lazy and would never amount to anything in life, let alone ever be able to take care of herself. And so far, her life lived up to this description. The result of these unchallenged and unexamined beliefs about herself has helped Sarah to have relationship after relationship with losers. So far, she's been in relationships only with drug addicts and emotional abusers.

Mary's parents believed their daughter's emotional sensitivity was abnormal. All of her life it was everyone's job to keep Mary happy so no one would have to contend with Mary's emotions. Even Mary's younger sister was put in charge of keeping Mary content to avoid what they deemed overly emotional responses.

Sixty years later, Mary believes she's too sensitive. She doesn't trust any of her feelings and only listens to others' interpretations of events. She doesn't even go to a movie unless her all-knowing sister says Mary will like the movie. Even worse than everyone telling Mary she's too sensitive, Mary believes them.

Being cut off from her emotional intelligence, Mary's life has brought her many stress-related physical illnesses and a lifetime of believing only others have the answers to life's questions. She gives little credence to her own opinion about anything. Not liking herself subtlety permeates every relationship and event in Mary's life. Coming closer to the end of her life, Mary is deeply sad, and in a marriage that's deteriorated into a not so peaceful coexistence.

Brad is 16 years old. During those 16 years his parents, who are inadequate and emotionally immature have contained their anxiety over managing life's tasks by controlling and manipulating everyone coming into their life, including their children. Brad's every behavior has been so controlled that a sense of autonomy and initiative have been completely stifled. He has no curiosity about the world and life. He has no life skills, is failing in school, and manages social relationships through intimidation and fights. He portrays an attitude of arrogance, but underneath all of his bravado is a scared and incompetent little boy. This sad little boy's body and mind is beginning to like girls, but there isn't a girl around that's interested in him. The disinterest of girls in Brad reinforces an already desperate view of himself.

Develop A Wonderful Relationship With Yourself

A great relationship is an outward manifestation of a great relationship with yourself. Trusting others starts with trusting yourself. Respect for others begins with respect for yourself. Here's how to develop a wonderful relationship with yourself by getting your head straight.

Develop The Tool Of Self-Awareness

Self-awareness is probably the most helpful tool that exists in your life. With self-awareness you benefit from knowing how you think and feel about what happens in your life. The more you know about yourself, the more information you have for making choices. Self-awareness means you know what, why, and when you choose whatever you do in your life.

Notice yourself. Pay attention to what you say and do and how you feel. Stop. Watch and listen to yourself. What do you see? What do you hear? Check in with yourself periodically, all day long, everyday. Stand outside of yourself and watch how you handle yourself and your life.

Paying attention to what you think and feel gives you valuable information for assessing your environment, other people, and choosing what or what not to do.

You may notice when you begin to pay closer attention to yourself that you can't always tell how you feel or what you think about something. When that happens to you, pause and take some time to listen to yourself. How do you think someone else may feel about what's happening? Are you so used to thinking and believing you feel like someone else says you should think or feel, that you've lost touch with how the real you thinks and feels? You are not anyone else you've ever known. You are equipped with your own senses that give you constant feedback. Listen to your own thoughts and feelings. Give your thoughts and feelings at least as much weight, as you would give someone else's opinions. Ideally, you'll count your own thoughts and feelings more heavily, unless the other person is an expert in the field in which they're offering you information. Even then, experts sometimes get stuck in what they read somewhere, rather than evaluating for themselves. Many experts believe that if they haven't read something somewhere, it can't be so.

You are the only real expert in your life. Pay attention to yourself.

During Carolyn's career she's worked

with some seriously dangerous mentally disturbed individuals. Doing so gave her an opportunity to learn to listen to herself like she had never listened before. In such a situation you must rely on your senses to guide your behavior or end up in some life threatening circumstances.

But trusting her own perceptions was difficult for Carolyn. It took several experiences with dangerous people to alert her to how trustworthy her perceptions were. One such case was a 16-year-old boy, hospitalized because of emotionally disturbed behavior, to which Carolyn never gave an inch. One day her supervisor reprimanded her for being so tough on this boy. Carolyn explained why she believed only rigid enforcement of the rules would benefit this boy. The supervisor didn't buy her explanation and Carolyn was scolded more. Three years later, Carolyn was reading the local paper and learned that this same boy, now 19, was apprehended after a random shooting spree with a shotgun. Three people had been killed as he drove up and down a local highway. Carolyn's trust in her perceptions grew.

Carolyn was the benefactor of so many of these kinds of experiences she became quite skillful at trusting her own perceptions. She was rarely wrong, even though all of her life others had attempted to dissuade her from what she knew. People were always trying to talk her out of what she saw and heard. And she struggled to hang on to some sense of trust in her perceptions. Carolyn became known in professional circles for recognizing dangerous individuals quickly, within a few minutes, compared to the months of repeated experiences it took others to recognize the truth.

Where did Carolyn get this information that eluded others so readily? From listening to herself. How did she learn to listen to herself so skillfully? From the brutal honesty with which she confronted her own and others' behaviors.

Fortunately, most people don't have to depend on these skills to save their lives literally. But less extreme examples happen all of the time. And saving your life from a bad marriage is every bit as life saving as saving yourself from a dangerous person. The only difference between a slow death and a quick death is the agony in-between.

Suzanne, from our previous example, was skillful at numbing her feelings. Initially, numbing herself served to prevent conflict, which she viewed as bad. But eventually, numbing herself led to lack of sexual desire and arousal. If Suzanne would have trusted her perceptions and listened to herself in the first place, she would have never married a man she didn't even like. Listening to herself would have given Suzanne the information she needed to make such an important decision.

Darlene hadn't been paying attention to herself from the beginning of her relationship with Tom. That is, she hadn't been listening until Tom beat her up one night. Darlene couldn't understand how she got herself mixed up with such a character, but it didn't take long to identify the clues that had been strewn about all along the way. Clues Darlene never acknowledged.

Several times Tom told Darlene to be quiet or he'd beat the stuffing (crap was his word) out of her. Darlene told herself he was teasing. After being stood up for a date, Tom told Darlene never to tell him what to do again, when she let him know how upset she was over being stood up. Tom and Darlene would have several fun dates and suddenly Tom disappeared for weeks at a time. Then he'd call and pick up with Darlene as nothing had happened.

If Darlene would have listened to herself – listened to her thoughts and feelings – she could have prevented being beaten by staying out of a relationship with a dangerous person.

Likewise, listening to yourself can tune you into the perfect marriage partner. Lynn was dating several young men. She wanted to get married and start a family soon. She was leaning toward marriage to Doug more than the others. But Lynn was chronically unhappy in the relationship. She kept trying to make their relationship work. At the same time she had a male friend, Stan, that she'd been a best friend with for several years. They had so much fun together, which was quite a contrast to her time with Doug. Every time she brought up Stan she glowed; when she talked about Doug she moaned and groaned, cried, yelled, and cursed. When Lynn learned to listen to herself she realized whom she should and shouldn't marry, and happily married Stan.

The Question Is: Who Are You?

Owning the parts of yourself that fit what you believe is good is usually much easier than owning the parts of yourself that fit what you believe is bad. Although, for some people, admitting they have good parts is more difficult than seeing themselves as bad. The truth is, we all have good and bad about us. Which parts of yourself do you freely admit to having? What about you do you avoid knowing?

Determination to know the real you is what it takes to begin to know all of the parts of yourself. Start by committing yourself to owning the real you.

Next, make two lists: include in the first list all of those things about yourself of which you like and approve. Include on the second list all of those things about yourself that you don't approve or like. Look over the lists and decide whether the lists are honest and reasonable. Are the good qualities over-inflated? Are there few good qualities that you can name? Are the so-called bad qualities really bad qualities? According to whom? Are there few to no bad qualities that you can identify?

One of the things you can do if your lists seem sparse or unrealistic is imagine what others would say are your good and bad qualities? You'll have to weigh and judge the accuracy of what another person would say, but what they say will give you a starting point for considering yourself. Yes, we said judge. You must make judgments constantly in life.

One of the best ways you can take a look at good or bad qualities you may be overlooking about yourself is to take a careful look at what you say about others. We often assign qualities to other people that are really qualities of ourselves that we have a much easier time identifying in someone else. Assigning those qualities to someone else is called projection. Sometimes the other person really does have elements of those qualities within themselves; if so, the person is mirroring qualities you have back to you. Sometimes the other person isn't even doing what you claim they're doing. In that case, the other person is merely acting as a blank piece of paper on which you paint yourself.

We all use projection to some degree. Some of us use it much more than others. We have a much easier time seeing parts of ourselves in someone else, than owning the qualities ourselves. The more you project, the more you disown aspects of yourself. Only when you develop a serious commitment to knowing the real you – good and bad – can you decrease projecting yourself onto someone else. Honesty about who you really are is the remedy for projection. And your task is to know the real you. In this case, we're recommending you use your projections to help you know yourself better.

Practice Self-Acceptance

To admit to having the parts of yourself for

which you don't approve, you must practice self-acceptance. Self-acceptance does not mean approving inappropriate behavior. Self-acceptance means realizing that you're human like the rest of us, and being open to the reality of who you are. You must allow yourself to know the parts of yourself of which you don't approve in order to make a decision about what to do. How can you change something you don't allow yourself to know about?

Andrea's relationships were riddled with arguments and conflict. She didn't realize that her tone of voice sounded angry all of the time – even when she wasn't angry. People were constantly misinterpreting her behavior; her relationships never lasted long. When someone pointed out to her that she sounded angry most of the time, asking Andrea if she was angry with them at that time, Andrea came into contact with an aspect about herself that she'd disowned to this point. From that moment forward Andrea's awareness of this tendency to sound angry opened her to changing her behavior. When she caught herself sounding angry she learned to apologize, saying she wasn't angry. Gradually, she learned to soften her tone. She learned to use words that sounded neutral rather than antagonistic.

When you have the opposite problem, not being able to own the good qualities about yourself, you can apply the same tactics to learn what they are. Listen to what others say are your good qualities. Listen to what you say when you recognize good qualities in others. Both activities can give you information about your own good qualities. People project their good qualities as well as their bad qualities onto others at times.

Tony met compliments with doubts they could really be true. In fact, Tony was a very bright person, talented in real estate development. His estimation about himself constantly underestimated his creativity, compassion, and sensitivity to social and business relationships. He had a gift for putting together real estate deals. But he had a hard time believing he was anything out of the ordinary.

Tony started listening to the compliments he gave others. Without too much trouble he began to appreciate that the very things he held in high regard about others were traits he had himself. He gradually came to humbly appreciate himself in a new light.

A slightly different situation, many people don't disbelieve compliments they get, but just don't know how to receive them. People discount the compliment with a mistaken response of self-effacement. When you mistakenly discount the compliment you miss the opportunity to learn something about yourself. If receiving compliments is uncomfortable for you because you don't know what to say, all you have to do is simply say, "thank you".

One caution: just as you may be describing yourself when you describe another person, when you listen to what someone says about you, they may really be describing themselves when they tell you what they see in you. Deciding what's accurate necessitates your thinking about, weighing, and judging what the person says. Do you do what the other person says you do? Or, have you noticed that the other person does exactly what they say you do?

If you can identify anyone in your life that you believe you can trust, ask him or her directly what they believe are your good and bad qualities. Asking others is tricky because other people project to some degree – some more or less than others. Only ask someone who seems to accept who you are without needling you to change. People that suggest you change are interested in accomplishing their own agenda, which may not take your agenda into consideration. Also, people have a tendency to see what they want to see, not necessarily what's really happening. But safe people exist. If you look carefully you may be able to identify a safe person from which you can learn much about yourself.

When George asked his brother how he saw George as a worker at the company where they both worked, his brother, Steve, said he thought George should work longer hours to get ahead and prove himself a loyal employee. To Steve, George's work behavior – eight-hour workdays – demonstrated disinterest.

That might have been important for George to know about himself, except that his brother works too much. Steve has a bad marriage and to avoid conflict and maintain the appearance of a good husband he spends many hours at work. It's true he's been rewarded with some promotions and raises George may never have, but what Steve deems as good work behavior is in the context of his avoidance of intimacy. You have to think for yourself and weigh the information you get.

Whereas, in the example with Andrea, Andrea obtained valuable and accurate information about her angry tone that helped her improve her relationship skills and know herself better.

How Does the Real You Compare with Who You Want to Be (Your Ideal You)?

Evaluate the marriage between the real you and your ideal you. Does who you want to be bicker with the real you? Bring the real you into line with the ideal you.

Jennifer wanted to have more courage to act honestly in her relationships. More and more she realized that, even though she had her own opinions about life and the world, she rarely stuck her neck out to express her own opinion. She admired a new friend of hers that spoke right up about what she believed. Her friend never seemed to mind that others argued their points with her, or put her down for not agreeing with their opinion. Her friend didn't seem afraid at all, that others would disapprove and not like her. In fact, Jennifer's friend seemed energized by expressing herself. Her energy and enthusiasm appealed to Jennifer. Jennifer wanted to be like her friend. Jennifer wanted to stop nagging herself to keep quiet, lest she alienate others.

Arnie wanted to live differently than in

the community where he grew up. The community is largely blue-collar workers whose lives change little from generation to generation. Arnie dreamed of a college education, flying his own plane, and a great marriage with the perfect partner. Arnie longed for an intimate relationship of equal partners that enjoyed a robust sex life. Slowly, he realized his mother was right. Arnie would have to leave this community in order to realize his dreams. Staying would mean spending most of his time and energy on defending his way of looking at life. Staying would mean only having the women within his own community from which to choose as a marriage partner.

For several years in late adolescence into young adulthood, Arnie heard what his mother said, he understood intellectually that to live the life he wanted he would have to live elsewhere. But he continued to stay. Finally, after one more bad relationship, Arnie connected emotionally with the idea of leaving. He started to plan a move that would take him into a location that fit with the realization of his dreams. He stopped fighting his dream.

For as long as Lisa could remember she'd wanted to be a nurse. The drama and glamour of work in a hospital, the idea of helping others, and catching a doctor husband all seemed like a great way to live. When Lisa got into nursing she slowly realized that nursing wasn't anything like what she'd imagined. Many of the people in the hospital she imagined helping substituted medical care for intimacy and caring in their relationships with friends and mates. Nice

and eligible doctors were few and far between.
For several years Lisa denied how unhappy she
felt from day to day. She constantly made excuses for staying, and stifled her yearning to find
more appealing work. Lisa kept looking for a
husband in a group of men that doesn't have
many men looking for loving and intimate marriages, with partner equality. Lisa spent her
time and energy forcing herself to behave in
conformity with her chosen profession.

One day, after being mistreated by one
more patient, and screamed at by one more
arrogant doctor, Lisa said enough is enough.
She decided to break out of the hostile shelter
she'd created through mistaken beliefs. She
decided she wanted to live in a way that
matched her much better than the world of
nursing. Lisa started listening to herself.

Andrea imagined herself to be compas-
sionate and understanding. The angry tone she
learned she displayed didn't fit with the image
she had of herself. She consciously worked on
changing her tone and vocabulary to fit the caring and friendly person she knew she was.

Robert alienated most women he dated.
He never seemed to be able to get past the first
date or two. In examining his interactions he
discovered that when he felt hurt he demonstrated anger and hostility. His demeanor was
rough and intimidating. He confronted his fear
of expressing hurt, learned that expressing hurt
didn't necessarily mean he was less of a man,
and gradually trusted himself to disclose the
real Robert. Changing his interactions in relationships opened the way for the women he

dated to have more honest and intimate exchanges with him. Robert liked the difference.

After you have what you consider to be an accurate list of good and bad qualities, you must make a decision about whether the qualities are good or bad because they are really good or bad, or because someone has been telling you all of your life those qualities are good or bad. You must decide for yourself. Go through and think about each quality.

Take some time to congratulate yourself for the qualities that you have that fit what you consider ideal and the list of good characteristics that really are good. Feel ownership. You can call on this list whenever you need to reality check the real you.

Joel's family had the habit of calling him selfish whenever Joel didn't do exactly what they wanted. The idea was to evoke guilt so he'd do what they wanted. After Joel worked on getting a clear picture of who he really is versus what he's been told repeatedly about himself, he had a tool with which to meet the guilt trips head on. With a clear and honest appraisal of himself and who he was, Joel just reminded himself of who he really was every time a family member dumped a guilt trip in his lap.

Consider the qualities you believe really are bad. Can any of them be changed? What would you like to exchange them for? Do you know anyone who demonstrates the ideal quality? If so, watch them. Imitate them. Teach yourself what to do instead. Read a book or magazine articles that describe what you'd like to change and follow their suggestions. Once you acknowledge what you dislike about yourself, usually the only thing that stands between what you want to be and who you are is failing to seek resources for change.

Consider Sarah, in our earlier example. For years her easygoing manner had been deemed laziness. She believed she was lazy; she never even considered the advantages of her low-keyed approach to life. If Sarah really were lazy, she'd benefit from finding out why she doesn't have any energy. Is she depressed? Is there something physically wrong? Or is this so-called laziness really just a different style of managing life? Or maybe non-action is the only way to wrestle control of her life from others.

In Sarah's case, her behavior was a combination of factors. Yes, she had an undiagnosed thyroid disorder. She actually had Grave's Disease, a thyroid condition that fluctuated between under function and over function. Many years of her life included constant readjustment to whatever state her thyroid was in. In combination with her physical condition, Sarah had a naturally calm and methodical approach to life. In comparison to her father's driven energetic style, Sarah's behavior seemed lazy. But lazy wasn't the right word for Sarah's behavior and believing she was lazy had negatively influenced everything she ever did.

Once you've identified good and bad qualities about yourself, you must pay attention to what in life fits the real you. Your likes and dislikes are important. Some are more negotiable than others are. Needs and wants are two different things. Needs are non-negotiable; wants are more or less negotiable.

Make one list that describes your needs and another list that describes your wants. One need is just as important as another is, but you can prioritize your wants. Decide how negotiable each want is. Be sure your needs and wants are your own needs and wants, not what someone else says should be your needs and wants.

Use the list in the next chapter, Differences That Make a Difference, to deepen the knowledge you have of yourself in regard to each characteristic. Describe who you are and what you believe for each characteristic.

Wes had difficulty differentiating his needs and wants from his parents'. It's common in his parents' generation to seek safety, stability, and security from work. Members of their generation sought employment that would last an adult lifetime. Because they sought to satisfy their needs and wants, Wes's parents achieved the kind of life style that provided financial safety, stability, and security. Because the household ran so smoothly, Wes automatically created a modern day version of their life style.

Unfortunately, the kinds of work that provide safety, stability, and security often provide a hefty measure of boredom. They rarely provide the opportunity for innovation. They rarely reward challenges to the status quo. Creative thought and innovative application of his knowledge energized Wes.

Initially Wes thought he wanted to be a

teacher or professor in a university. His first wife wanted to be a teacher and liked the idea of the life style attached. She was content to support herself at the level of survival. The idea of living the life of teachers contributed to their illusion of compatibility. Since Wes had the idea to be a teacher stemming from the safe, stable, and secure life of his parents, and the career didn't fit the real Wes, it wasn't long before he failed, and changed his mind about that career path. His next career choice fit him better; it used some of his intelligence, but no where near his capabilities. The closer Wes got to discover the real Wes, the more he differed from his first wife's idea of a good husband.

Make Sure You Have a Good Reputation with Yourself

One of the biggest reasons people choose someone with many differences is that they want to make up for characteristics for which they believe they're lacking. If you pick someone as a partner who makes up for your deficiencies, the relationship is a set-up for power struggles and mutual disapproval from the beginning. Instead, be the way you want your partner to be. Learn how to do life tasks yourself. Become independent so you don't need someone to take up the slack. Being able to handle life's tasks enables give and take in a marriage. Independence is the forerunner to interdependence. Interdependence is the style of interaction that works the best in relationships. Interdependence is necessary for a great marriage.

In a marriage between interdependent adults, both partners can handle most anything that confronts them. They may be better or worse at some things, but in the final wash, both partners are either able to handle the task themselves, or know how to seek appropriate resources to learn or delegate the task.

There is only one way for you to feel good about yourself. To earn a good reputation with yourself you must take responsibility for your life, be competent, and live with integrity. Feeling good about yourself comes from trusting your own perceptions and from trusting yourself to handle life.

Be Competent

Handle tasks of daily living consistently. If you don't know how to do something, learn. Since there just isn't time to be good at everything, delegate tasks to appropriate resources in the community. Learn to balance your checkbook, follow a budget, shop for groceries, and wash your clothes. Find a comfortable style for doing tasks of daily living, that you can do without a partner. If you don't like to iron, budget for taking your shirts to the cleaner. If balancing a checkbook is a difficult chore, keep your checkbook on the computer and let software keep your budget and balance. No one right way exists to handle life. The point is to handle life yourself in a style that supports your values.

Being competent frees you to marry the right partner, not just any partner or someone that fills in your gaps.

Be Effective

Learn to discern the important in life from the unimportant in life. Set goals that fit the real you. Learn to achieve your goals. Decide what you want, break getting what you want down into manageable pieces, and consistently accomplish what you set out to do step-by-step. Learn the skills necessary to master each step of reaching your goal. If your relationship skills aren't what it takes to handle social situations, learn more about social skills. If you want to run your own business, decide what skills are necessary and learn them. Go back to school, read books and magazines, watch others. Set your life up to support you in getting what you want. Attend to your appearance. Blend your personal style with the requirements for the task.

Being effective liberates you to have what you want.

Earn Your Own Trust

Listen to what your own perceptions tell you. See what you see, hear what you hear. Believe what your senses say. You have what it takes to collect the information you need to manage your life. Your senses are as good as anyone else's.

Handle life rather than letting it handle you. Become accustomed to handling tasks of daily living on a regular basis to prevent crises. Taking care of business along the way stops life circumstances from jerking you around. Become a problem solver, a solutions expert. See obstacles as a challenge and move beyond them. Do whatever is necessary, now. Either you'll take the time and energy today, or twice the time and energy tomorrow, after the crisis.

Trusting yourself is the precursor to trusting others and others trusting you.

Act with Intention

When you live without thinking about what you're doing you're reacting. You're letting whatever happens now, or happened in the past, govern your response. Instead, stop and think first. Make whatever you do intentional, on purpose. Are you sure you've interpreted the events accurately? What are all of the possible interpretations? What options do you have in regard to your response? What are the potential outcomes of your options for behavior? It is possible to over-analyze, paralyzing yourself, but err on the side of thinking things over, rather than an immediate reaction.

Acting with intention helps you to feel

good about yourself, increases your competence and effectiveness, helps you solve problems and trust yourself, and dramatically increases your chances of getting what you want.

Live in the Here and Now

When you stop and think, you increase your ability to respond to the task at hand, and you decrease the possibility of your responding to an event from your past. Our brains categorize events, their causes and effects. Unless we stop and discern the current event and characters from the events and characters of our past, we end up responding as if we were in the past event. When you respond as you did in the past, or based on your past experience, you diminish your chance to respond appropriately now.

　　Living in the here and now allows you to design your behavior specifically for the current event. Designing your behavior specifically for the task at hand improves your ability to get the desired result.

Should You Get Your Head Straight on Your Own or in Therapy?

The process is similar no matter which you do, but some definite advantages exist for getting into therapy. Getting your head straight is a bit like peeling an onion. One layer gives way to the next. You can peel the layers of the onion on your own, but doing so is difficult for some of us to do. And some onions cause so many tears you can't see the onion to peel. Uncovering the layers can be difficult because exposing the past, how much your behavior differs from the real you, and how you feel about yourself causes varying amounts of pain and grief. Uncovering the real you does offer tremendous relief, like a weight being lifted from your shoulders, but having emotional support and an experienced guide helps to ease the confusion and pain and facilitates relief.

You can do the work of getting your head straight on your own. Books exist that can help you understand issues in your life, the unfinished business of your past, and whatever gets into your way of being who you really are, living competently and effectively, feeling good about yourself, trusting yourself, acting with intention, and living in the here and now. The ease with which you can accomplish getting your head straight varies from person to person. Obviously, the less trouble you have with the tasks to master, the better able you'll be at achieving maturity on your own.

Whether difficult or easy, definite advantages exist in therapy — at least, therapy with the right person. The right therapist is someone with whom you feel emotionally safe, but who isn't afraid to confront real issues for you. They know about the issues regarding events of your past that get in the way of knowing and being yourself, being competent and effective, trusting yourself, acting with intention, and living in the here and now. Pick a therapist that can tell you, generally, what they've done to heal him or herself. The therapist doesn't need to, and shouldn't, bare their soul to you, but be human enough to acknowledge they've worked through some of the same tasks. The therapist needs to be able to be honest and real with you. They need to be able to be direct in a friendly way, not afraid to confront you, demonstrating how to set limits and boundaries in a respectful way. The right therapist facilitates your competence and independence.

The biggest advantage to therapy is that a good therapist has the ability to point out connections you may miss. A good therapist lends objectivity to your examination and appraisal of you. Having the support and guidance of a good therapist can speed the process of becoming competent, effective, and independent. Being in therapy offers you an opportunity to experience yourself in a relationship where the therapist accepts the real you and validates your perception of events. Being in therapy offers you an opportunity to practice new behaviors before they count as much as they do in public.

Effective therapy can enhance and speed the process of finding the right partner for a great marriage.

For those of you who need therapy, but believe you can't afford it – we say you can't afford not to afford it! Much greater expense exists down the road if you don't invest in yourself right now. Divorces are expensive financially and emotionally. Children's emotional disorders are expensive. Frequent job changes and unhappy job experiences can be expensive. The emotional toll unhappiness takes on your life is much more expensive than therapy.

What you need to do to get your head straight is hard work. But this hard work doesn't compare at all to the heartache and pain marriage to the wrong partner creates. We guarantee that your commitment to getting your head straight will result in the skills necessary to find and create a great marriage. Every other thing you must do to have your own great marriage grows from the maturity and competence of getting your head straight.

5

16 Differences That Make a Difference

What to Look for in Your Perfect Partner

Clearly defining what you want is a process of bringing to awareness, naming, and picturing the characteristics and qualities of the person you want for your marriage partner and the kind of relationship you want. Clearly defining what you want replaces thoughtless action and reaction with intentional action. Intentional action increases your ability to be successful. Clearly defining what you want programs your sub-conscious mind to help you get what you want. When your sub-conscious mind has the same information that your conscious mind has, it can help you do subtle things in your everyday life to bring you what you want, rather than work against what you want, drawing to you the same mistakes over and over.

Clearly defining what you want began in the previous chapter where you got to know who you are in relation to the 16 Things To Know About Yourself. Review what you think and believe about the attributes on the list. If you didn't take time to think this through in chapter four, do it now. You must first know who you are. The way you think, believe, and feel about these characteristics helps to define who you are.

Next, pay particular attention to thinking about what kind of relationship you want. Knowing who you are includes knowing what you expect from your marriage. Different people want different things from their marriage. Just make certain that what you say you want is what you want, not something someone else has said you should want.

Describe what you've learned in writing. Keep a log (workbooks available – see order form at the back of this book or check your local bookstore). The picture of who you are and what you want will continue to evolve. Add details to the written description of who you are and what you want, as you become aware of them.

When you know what you think, believe, and feel about each attribute you'll know what characteristics and qualities about your partner fit you. And that's the key. On the 16 differences that make a difference you must match to a high degree.

Picture someone with those characteristics in your mind. Be aware of what kind of emotions arise about the person as well as the kind of marriage you want. Experiencing the emotions attached to your perfect partner and a great marriage increases the ability of your subconscious mind to help find them. A clear picture with emotion intensifies the ability to draw them to you.

Write down descriptions of your perfect partner for each of the 16 differences. Avoid writing what you think you want. Write what matches you. As you sift through the qualities and characteristics of people you date or meet, add detail to your written description.

Be sure to frame what you want in the context of what you want, not what you don't want. You'll get whatever you think about. If you think about what you don't want you'll get what you don't want. Whenever you notice yourself thinking or worrying about what you don't want, redirect your thoughts and refocus on what you do want.

You may not realize that getting what you want really is as easy as consciously naming what you want. The act of self-awareness and bringing to awareness your thoughts and feelings, itself, assists you in making your hopes and dreams come true. Be careful not to underestimate the value of consciousness. A vital key to leading the life you want lies in aligning unconscious and sub-conscious beliefs with what you consciously say you want.

Marie married an alcoholic. Having grown up in a household where no one drank and where most family members took life very seriously, Fred's fun loving, partying family was a welcome relief. Little did Marie know that, in reality, their carefree behavior was serious, pervasive alcoholism. Further into the marriage, after three children and many broken promises, Marie began to realize the extent of the problem and that she would most likely spend many years nursing a sickly husband in end-stage alcoholism. Or lose him altogether. She felt heartsick realizing the genetic and behavioral legacy her children had been handed.

Marie endured eight years of increasing awareness of the extent and seriousness of her mate's drinking problem. Becoming more aware, Marie developed intense anxiety about what would become of her. She began to see how dependent she was herself on having a mate. A dependency that prevented her from acting upon the sense that the healthiest thing to do would be to end the marriage. Eight years of fighting to change her husband's behavior, therapy, and worry about what would become of her and the children finally pushed Marie over the edge. She had to save herself and hopefully the children.

So Marie left the marriage after eighteen years. Unfortunately, she focused on what she didn't want. She didn't want another mate who had a problem with alcohol. She didn't spend any time focused on what she did want; she neglected to bring to awareness not only that she wanted a mate that didn't drink, but also a mate that had matured into a competent adult. She hadn't realized that a drinking problem often prevents the drinker from learning more constructive behaviors; she didn't think through what level of competence she wanted her mate to have; she didn't think through what actions would match competent and effective behavior. She just knew she didn't want to be alone and afraid.

A few years later Marie married again. Within three and a half years her new husband died. His heavy chronic drinking contributed to his inability to fight a devastating infection. At the age of forty she found herself widowed – alone and afraid. She got exactly what she worried about.

Without going into all of the details, suffice it to say that Marie got serious about figuring out how to find a compatible and competent mate. She spent a year of concentrated effort to teach herself how to take charge of her life and get what she wanted. She didn't date anyone during that time. She couldn't afford to get distracted from finishing her own unfinished business. She followed the process outlined in this book. She learned to focus on what she wanted, not what she didn't want. And it worked. She found the perfect mate for herself and has a great marriage. She made her hopes and dreams come true.

How Did We Decide On This List of Characteristics?

This list of characteristics – of differences that

make a difference – has been distilled from: our own experiences with the wrong mates; the experience of family, friends, and hundreds of patients; the role model of Carolyn's son's great marriage; a close examination of why our great marriage is so wonderfully different from others; and lists of characteristics and qualities that other professionals have created. The following is the sequence of events that led us to the creation of the differences that make a difference.

Both of us came out of our previous marriages knowing what we didn't want. As a first step, knowing what we didn't want certainly helped but still didn't give us a clear picture of what to aim for instead. As well as her own marriage, Carolyn had fifteen years of experience working with individuals, couples, and families in her practice. Her professional experience reinforced all of the issues in broken relationships. Knowing what didn't work for others and us highlighted certain categories of problems predominating in problem marriages, thereby giving us a start on our list. We both had the hope for a great marriage. Neither of us wanted to believe poor and mediocre marriages were the only kinds of marriages in existence. We both had the determination to learn and grow. But neither of us had had the benefit of seeing a great marriage in operation – not a single role model. That is, until Carolyn had the privilege of watching one of her sons fall in love.

Nine years ago, Ryan fell in love with Amanda one summer between college semesters. Amanda had a summer job where Ryan and many of his friends worked. Her school semester ended sooner than Ryan's; she arrived at her summer job ahead of him. Many of Ryan's friends were already there for the summer – friends he'd had since elementary and junior high school. They all liked Amanda. What's ironic is that they all also agreed that Amanda was Ryan's type, and they'd wait to ask her out to see if he liked her first.

Ryan and Amanda liked each other immediately. They started to date and became really good friends. To make a long story short, they fell in love and married three years later. Their friendship and love has supported them each in graduating from college, getting their first postgraduate jobs, quitting their jobs to return to graduate school, and graduating with an MBA and a Law degree. They've gotten jobs and live exactly where they want to be.

These two are a joy to be around. The energy they generate has supported them in setting and achieving the life goals of which they've dreamed. The energy from their marriage gave Carolyn what she was looking for: an example of an extraordinary great marriage, which provided the target for which to aim.

The difference between all of the poor and mediocre marriages and this great marriage were the differences or similarities of certain characteristics between partners.

Going to a national dating service provided the next step for each of us in honing the list of characteristics. (We know dating services have gotten some bad press, but hear us out. We had a great experience. The dating service gave us, as busy working professionals, dramatically more people to date than we would have had otherwise – and more).

To participate in the dating service we each had to fill out a profile that was housed in a notebook along with other members, each matched with pictures of the member. The profiles were one page packed with information about the member designed to inform other members about enough to determine potential compatibility. The top half of the profile provided demographic information like the city the member lived in, height, weight, birth date, occupation, education, where raised, marital status, whether you smoke or drink, number of children, whether you wanted children, religious/spiritual affiliations, religious dating preference, and cultural dating preferences. The bottom half of the profile held answers to three topics: what you like to do, who you are, and what you're looking for.

As you might imagine, filling out our profiles forced us to clarify who we are and what we wanted. The information on the profile sharpened the list of specific characteristics for which to seek compatibility. During the process of identifying potential dates we were forced to focus on what we wanted.

When we realized what we'd found – the marriage of our dreams – we felt that others could benefit immensely from what we'd learned.

Next came two years of researching what others had written to date about marriage and relationships. We knew that after having good relationship skills and maturity that compatibility was the key. So we examined every list of characteristics that other professionals had written. What we found, though, were loosely structured, cumbersome lists, long and vague lists of characteristics, none of which offered a specific list of qualities and characteristics that you could use to measure your compatibility easily. In a few cases we found lists of the wrong things about a prospective partner, a buying list focused on undesirable qualities.

The following list of 16 differences that make a difference contains what we believe are the crux of compatibility. Our distilled list of specific characteristics is designed to enable you to focus directly of differences that mean a bad or mediocre marriage if you don't match or a great marriage if you do match.

Keep in mind that our aim is to have a great marriage, not just any marriage. You can make concessions on these characteristics, but the degree to which you do will decrease your chance for a great marriage. And remember all of the characteristics are equally important. Once again...

16 Differences That Make a Difference

1. Sexdrives/sexual interests/demonstration of affection
2. Age
3. Health and fitness, including the habits

of smoking, drinking, or using drugs
4. Where to live
5. Education/Intelligence
6. Lifestyle (Formal versus Informal)
7. Views about work/Level of ambition
8. Views on how to handle and spend money
9. Expectations of marriage/relationship
10. Physical characteristics attractive to you
11. Religious beliefs and practices
12. Political beliefs and practices
13. Children: Having them and raising them
14. Life stage
15. Common leisure interests
16. Energy levels

Differences That Make A Difference

We're not talking about just any kind of differences here. We're talking about differences that call into question someone's integrity.

Tolerance of human differences is a noble endeavor. In most areas of living, such as work and friendship, an appreciation for differences offers us a civil community in which to live and work. Appreciation of differences can contribute to the attainment of individual potential. When someone lives up to their highest potential they contribute positively to their social group and everyone benefits. When each individual operates at their highest ability the group of which they are part functions best. Seeing circumstances from another person's point of view offers you a wider perspective for satisfactory living. Many different ways of living are healthy and normal.

While you tolerate differences between you and your coworkers and friends, you're free to return home to live life in a way most satisfying to you. Not having to negotiate and compromise with coworkers and friends on every task of life saves your work relationships and friendships from conflict and exhaustion.

That is not so for married couples. Marriage intensifies differences because of proximity. Differences that make a difference cause children to choose loyalty between two parents along with learning values.

Mary won a trip for two to Hollywood to participate in the taping of a popular TV show. Her husband couldn't go because of work so Mary decided to take a friend of hers from school. They'd become good friends over the past two years, studying and socializing together often. Being with each other twenty-four hours a day for five days was an entirely different matter. They never wanted to do the same activities. Every decision resulted in compromise and disappointment. Exhaustion best describes how Mary felt on her return.

Marriage is not the place to learn to tolerate differences. A high level of compatibility between marriage partners on the following 16 characteristics are a requirement for a great marriage.

For every single characteristic on this list

of important differences, each of you has a right to your own feelings and beliefs. Unless your behavior infringes upon the rights of others, you have a right to behave in keeping with your feelings and beliefs. With this in mind, let's take a look at the 16 differences that make a difference – this time in relation to describing your perfect partner. A high level of attunement on these potential similarities or differences between you and your partner is the key to a great marriage.

Sex Drive/ Sexual Interests/ Displays of Affection

How often does your partner like to have sex? Is your partner adventuresome or do they like a tried and true routine? Do they like to hold hands? How do they feel about kissing in public? What kinds of behaviors tell them they're loved and appreciated? What displays of affection are they comfortable with in front of your children?

Individuals differ in the amount of sex they want, differ in their patterns of arousal, and differ in their desire for displays of affection. But, all humans want sex and affection to some degree. The level of difference in drive for sexual satisfaction and the level of desire for affection between individuals fit into a wide range of normal behavior. Because a wide range of normal behavior exists, you must carefully match yourself to a partner of equal drive and desire.

He Said

I enjoy sex. I have a high sex drive and like to express affection freely. Nothing reassures me more about myself and my love relationship than frequent sexual expression. I like to satisfy my partner. Part of my arousal comes from exciting my partner.

My first wife had a much lower sex drive than I had. Once she had the two children she wanted and stopped accommodating to my desires, sex in our marriage dwindled to a negotiated twice a week. Sex twice a week seemed like starvation to me; sex twice a week was far too much for my former wife.

My first wife and I divorced largely because of extremely different ideas about our sexual relationship and expectations of marriage.

On the other hand, Carolyn and I match well on sexual drive, desire, and displays of affection. The behaviors that come naturally to each of us are so comfortable to the other that negotiation isn't necessary. Instead of being a source of friction between us, our trust, affection for each other, and intimacy are deepened by our sexual relationship.

She Said

Sex is also a big deal to me. I like sexual expression; I'm affectionate and demonstrative. During my life I've met many men, in my personal life and as a therapist or friend, who felt seriously inconvenienced by changing their sexual routine to satisfy their partner. They believed something must be wrong with their partner if they couldn't have an orgasm from intercourse. I've also met men who had low sex drives that informed me that something must be wrong with me or their partner because all I or their partner ever thought about was sex. They actually believed women weren't supposed to like sex.

Meeting someone who matched me sexually, that was interested in pleasuring and satisfying me the way I like and need to be pleasured, was a wonderful relief. Wes's desire to satisfy me deepens my trust in and affection for him. Having Wes welcome the loving expressions I have to offer is like getting a gift.

Reconciling yourself to a slight difference may not be stressful, but anything bordering on deprivation or force is unacceptable. Mismatched sex drives can cause a shift in the balance of power in marriage. The partner who doesn't need or want sex so much gains power over the other by giving them sex. Differences in this area are so stressful they cause deep dissatisfaction and resentment, infidelity, and divorce.

Age

What kind of music does your partner like? What events transpired during his or her life that influences their values? An example would be having lived through the depression or the sixties and those events having influenced how they spend and save money, how they feel about war, how they feel about establishment mores. What does your partner believe about the roles of husbands and wives?

Differences in your age with a mate matter more or less depending on how old you are. When you're 16 to 30 a small age difference can make a huge difference in what you're doing in life, and how you enjoy life. During this time, major differences exist in levels of maturity. People mature at different rates. People also enjoy activities related to their generation.

As you reach 30, a few years difference in age makes less of a difference. With compatible levels of maturity, people with a few years of difference in age can still enjoy compatibility in other aspects of their life.

Many years of difference in age matter often enough to prevent compatibility in many of the other characteristics on which you must match for any hope of a great marriage.

Roger is 50 and Sally is 28. Roger feels proud that he attracted such a young and beautiful mate; Sally feels secure with an older man. Unfortunately, as soon as the initial sexual attraction settled into married life, they began to notice their differences. Sally wanted children and all of the attending life style. She looked forward to driving the kids to ball games and other childhood activities. She wanted to participate in PTA and community endeavors.

Roger wanted to slow down. He'd had three children in his first marriage. He didn't think having one or two more children with Sally would be a big deal, but he began to dread all of the work involved. He'd just reached a stage in his life where the kids could do a lot for themselves; he realized more children meant paying college tuition far longer than he'd anticipated.

Sally also started feeling Roger was a real drag on her social life. She liked to go out and party with friends frequently; Roger liked reading and listening to music at home. And Sally despised the music Roger liked. When they got together with friends, either one or the other had fun, not both.

Of the 16 differences that make a difference, twelve can be seriously affected because of an age difference. Pick a partner within a few years of your age one way or the other. Only if you match well on every other characteristic on our list with a prospective partner, and then, only if you can answer yes to the other four important questions (chapter 8) should you even consider someone of a greater age difference than just a few years.

Health and Fitness, Including the Habits of Smoking, Drinking, or Using Drugs

How does health and fitness affect your partner's lifestyle? What do they practice in their life in relation to health and fitness? What do they do to maintain their health? Notice their beliefs and feelings about diet, exercise, rest and relaxation. How do they want you to fit into their practices?

Our interest here is to help you realize how important the issues surrounding health and fitness are to your overall happiness and, more specifically, your satisfaction and happiness in your marriage. And health and fitness are vital to great sex and your attractiveness in the dating marketplace, as well as, your overall ability to function constructively in everyday life.

Smoking, drinking, and using drugs each affect your life style. Now you may be tempted to hear this as judgmental, but these health issues aren't moral issues – they're issues concerning your health, the health of your mate, and the health of future children. Each affect health and fitness. The social lives of people that use cigarettes, cigars, pipes, alcohol, and or drugs usually revolve around their use. Your or your partner's use or non-use of these substances models behavior for your children and will affect their health and well being. Smoking, drinking alcohol, and using drugs can each affect children before and after birth. Decisions – judgments – in this case are necessary if you want to find the right mate to marry.

Obviously, if you're a smoker, you'll match better with a smoker. If you drink alcohol, you'll match better with someone who drinks alcohol. The same for using drugs. This book is about finding the right mate for a great marriage. You have to match, but you also have to function at your healthiest and most mature level to achieve what we're talking about. A great marriage takes both compatibility and mental and physical health.

When Roseanne married Jason it never occurred to her Jason's smoking, drinking and occasional marijuana use would cause a problem in their marriage. He didn't use them much and he was usually considerate about when and how much he smoked and drank. However, when Roseanne was pregnant she began to notice how much Jason's use of these substances affected how she felt physically and emotionally. She worried about how second-hand smoke would affect the baby. She worried that Jason's being under the influence of alcohol or marijuana might compromise his behavior and somehow injure the baby. She worried the baby would grow up and use substances that might harm his or her health. She worried about the health of her husband, the father of their children.

Roseanne didn't want to sit in smoke filled rooms anymore. She didn't have fun anymore at parties where drinking and smoking marijuana occurred. Stale smoke made her feel sick.

Roseanne and Jason began to argue. Jason argued that Roseanne never objected before. He felt she was changing the rules in the middle of the game. He felt that Roseanne was trying to control everything he did and resented her disapproval. Jason had never had to consider how much his behavior impacted on others until now.

Roseanne appreciated that she'd changed her mind; she realized she did want to change the rules. But how could she know what a difference pregnancy and having children would make to her about the use of these substances? Jason didn't want to give up these behaviors;

Roseanne knew she couldn't admire someone who didn't take a helpless child's health and well being into consideration and stop habits that were harmful to all. How could she not care about her husband and children?

This argument escalated into a downward spiral from which Roseanne and Jason never recovered. Their new child's parents divorced when their daughter was six months old.

Where to Live

In what climates would your partner be happy to make their home? Does distance from their family and friends affect where they want to live? Do local politics mesh with their beliefs? Does it matter if they move around? Do they have any allergies that would make living somewhere miserable? What kind of recreational activities do they like? Do certain geographical areas support or hinder living life that way they want to live?

Where you live affects how you feel physically and emotionally. Climate and the presence of allergens (airborne pollens and molds that inhabit the area) affect different people different ways. If you spend most of your time and energy battling an environment hostile to your health, doing so will have a profound affect on your feelings toward a partner who stays healthy and fit in the same environment. Basically, you must both be able to maintain your health and comfort easily in the environment in which you choose to live.

Jim and Louise moved to upper state New York because Jim got promoted and transferred. Louise wasn't happy about the move to a colder climate, she's cold unless the temperature is eighty or above. Within months of their move, Louise faced a winter such as she'd never experienced before. She had the flu and numerous colds throughout the winter. In the spring she still felt cold and had allergic reactions to the tree pollen and grasses native to the area. For four short weeks in the summer Louise felt comfortable, healthy; she resumed her usual active social life. In the fall she felt miserable because of the cold dampness. The second winter she experienced more physical illness and Seasonal Affective Disorder (depression related to lack of sunlight); she became so depressed she couldn't make herself function from day to day.

Louise's discomfort had nothing to do with her love for her husband. But problems with her health did affect their relationship negatively. Jim loved his wife, but how could he give up the opportunity of a lifetime, the job he'd been working toward his entire career?

You may think the climate and temperature is a trite reason by which to choose a marriage partner, but if you spend your life cold all of the time, how long before your irritability affects the way you relate to others? And if your partner is hot all of the time and can't sleep, how long before their lethargy and irritability erodes their love for you? What if the only vacation you take during the year is to a place that's hostile to your well being? Let's say, to compensate you and your mate agree to alternate years that each can choose their vacation for the year. Can you tolerate only vacationing every other year in a climate you like, knowing your partner hates every moment? And taking separate vacations means not sharing fun, rest, and recreation with the person you love. Can you afford to associate only the work of life with your marriage?

Of course minor adjustments can be made by the use of more or less clothes, or taking allergy shots, or taking medicine, or even using lamps to prevent Seasonal Affective Disorder, but at what cost? Where do you draw the line? How much is it reasonably possible to change your body's reaction to the climate?

Distance between you and family and friends affects different people in different ways. Frequent moves satisfy the wanderlust in some people, but prevent stability and equilibrium in others. Moves offer promotion at work to some, but force others to start their own businesses over.

Tim loved new adventures. He looked forward to living in many different places. His wife, Jane, didn't care where they lived as long as it was no more than a mile from her mother. Tim believed Jane would change after marrying him; he believed their love would encourage her to want to travel around and be with him. The first time he pushed the issue, they moved and Jane tried to make new friends to replace the contact she'd always had with her parents. But it was more than Jane could handle. The anxiety and anguish caused by being away from her parents prevented Jane from being interdependent in her relationship with Tim and prevented her from transferring her loyalty to the new family unit she made with Tim. Their marriage ended with hurt feelings and a sense of failure for both.

Education/Intelligence

What does your partner like to talk about? Are they interested in current events or the latest science and technology? Do they like to discuss literature and film? Or would they rather focus their life on children and home? Do they surf the Internet? Is their favorite pastime watching sports on TV? What do they like to read? Does the kind of work they do influence their lifestyle? What do they think about going to college?

Remember here that you need to know who you really are. You need to act like the real you. You need to like the real you. How smart you are is part of the real you. Self-awareness leads to information about yourself that will help you match the right person. Self-acceptance leads to acting like and liking the real you. An accurate appreciation of your level of intelligence will help you choose the right person for a great marriage. Don't write off matching on level of intelligence because you feel offended by thinking about your and someone else's level of intelligence. More or less intelligence isn't inherently good or bad. Every level of intelligence has its good and bad points. Brutal honesty about your intelligence adds to your ability to find the right partner. If you're dishonest with yourself about this quality, if you pick someone smarter to balance less intelligence or someone not as smart (for a variety of reasons) you'll seriously impair your chance for a great marriage.

Your level of intelligence affects how you understand what happens in your life and the world, topics of conversation, and what you spend your time doing. Your level of intelligence influences your problem solving ability, and your problem solving style. Your level of intelligence influences your educational ambitions. Your level of intelligence helps to define your social circle. Your level of intelligence impacts on whether you and your partner can understand each other. Your level of intelligence influences whether you can talk to each other over breakfast.

Differences in levels of intelligence between people in work and community groups are more easily tolerated than within a marriage because of less intense interaction and less time spent together. Also, dependence on the adequate function of the group is spread out between many people.

In a marriage equal levels of intelligence contribute to your ability to work and play together as a team. Equality balances power. In a marriage the family depends on two adults to carry the load.

Meg married Stan. Stan was a great guy, he worked hard, participated in community affairs, but he was a plain and simple guy with an average intelligence. Meg felt tremendous attraction to Stan; they had lots of physical chemistry. She especially loved his boyish charm. Stan was dependable and loyal, but Meg could never discuss many of her interests with Stan. Meg enjoyed contemplating life and exploring abstract ideas; doing so stimulated her. Whenever Meg tried to engage Stan in such conversations, Stan became quickly impatient. He just couldn't understand why Meg had to think so deeply, or make such a big deal out of something that seemed so simple to him. When problems arose they had even more trouble. Stan was easily frustrated by challenge, most often avoiding anything that might require problem solving. He'd rather just go along smoothly, living from day to day without rocking the boat. Meg never met an obstacle she didn't see as a challenge. She engaged in life without regard for problems that might arise. She had a lifetime of experiences that had taught her she could learn to handle new tasks or easily find someone who could. She loved the challenge of growth and change.

Needless to say, their excitement for each other quickly wore thin. Stan was increasingly threatened by anything Meg might say that he couldn't understand. Meg felt bored. She felt she had to walk on eggshells lest she cause Stan frustration. The choices they have are to go on and live increasingly separate lives; a life where Meg concedes never to expect too much from her marriage; a life of turning outside her marriage for intellectual stimulation. In such a situation, Stan would have to find companionship with others. Stan would have to accept that he'd never be able to provide intellectual companionship to his wife. Or, to try and get someone to change. But how do you change intelligence? And yet another choice is to leave the marriage. None of the choices can possibly engender a great marriage.

For a great marriage you must select a partner with a similar level of intellectual ability.

Educational level is easier to change than intelligence, but still lends itself to a wide range of possibilities. Educational drive and achievement contribute to a marriage's life style, interests and activities. Formal pursuits of education often contribute to how much time and energy someone has for a relationship, and therefore can contribute to expectations partners have of their marriage.

Differences in educational ambition and achievement encourage an imbalance of power between partners.

A common example that most of you have seen at some point in your life is what happened to Joanne and George. Having been high school sweethearts, they married a year after high school graduation. That year had given Joanne an opportunity to work and to save some money and for George to finish a year of college.

They moved into married housing on a large university campus. Joanne worked full time as an office manager in a small insurance company. She also took care of the small apartment and kept track of their social calendar. Life was wonderful in the beginning, but by

George's second year of medical school Joanne was tired of supporting them. She wanted to stay home and have a couple of children. She felt more and more out of place at the social activities they attended. She didn't have anything to say to George's friends. George never had time to spend with Joanne and her friends. What's more, George never had much to say to her anymore.

George felt angry about this change in Joanne. He couldn't believe she'd withdraw her support toward his educational and career goals. She'd always been proud of his wanting to be a doctor. Lately, he perceived Joanne as being a real drag on him; increasingly, she couldn't relate to his ideas, interests, or his ambition.

Joanne felt George only thought of himself. His reaction to her attempts to compromise increased the friction. Joanne thought George should interrupt medical school, take a break and work for a few years so Joanne could have children. Joanne just didn't understand that such an interruption could cost George his dream of becoming a doctor. She even thought that not becoming a doctor would improve their social lives. More and more she resented spending the money she made on George's dreams. She lost interest in sex. If George couldn't give Joanne what she wanted, then she wasn't going to give George what he wanted. After all, how could she have sex with someone who treated her as hired help?

Initially George chose to stick with school, but tried to spend more time with

Joanne. That choice didn't meet with Joanne's idea of compromise. She continued to nag George to leave school. Afraid he might lose Joanne he finally left school. He didn't realize he'd already lost Joanne. Now his choice would cause his losing himself and his dream.

Work was agony for George. He felt stifled and trapped. Joanne busied herself with her new baby, rarely spending any time with her husband. His resentment grew. Their conflict escalated to divorce.

When you ask someone to give up their dream, you ask them to compromise their integrity. Psychological health mandates the maintenance of integrity. You should get into a war to the end – power struggles – when your integrity is at stake.

Wendy stuck it out in her marriage to Richard. She marveled at his graduation from law school. She overlooked their differences in friendships and social circles, her inability to relate to his work world and philosophical ideas. She felt good about herself and her role as homemaker, mother, and wife. Proud that she'd supported her man, Joanne had helped Richard to attain his educational goals.

His marriage bored Richard. Home and companionship with Wendy tortured him. He began to feel embarrassed about Wendy when attending social functions related to his work or his friendships. Richard depended more and more on other relationships to satisfy his desire for social, intellectual, and emotional companionship. Richard fell in love with a fellow attorney. He divorced Wendy within a year and a half of his graduation from law school. Enraged, Wendy couldn't understand how Richard could leave her after she'd actually helped him get what he wanted.

When you make compromises about your life it doesn't work. It didn't work when Joanne pushed the issue with George; it didn't work when Wendy supported her man.
Lifestyle

Lifestyle is a way of life that reflects your attitudes and values.

Does your partner like to live casually or do they prefer a more formal way of life? Are they a morning or a night person? Are they active or inactive? Would they rather be outdoors or indoors? How active are they socially? What kind of house do they want to live in, and in what neighborhood? How do they want to furnish their house? What kind of food do they like, meat and potatoes, gourmet dining, or perhaps vegetarian? How do they like to spend mealtime?

Mary believes that your home is the one place in the world where you can let down your hair and put your feet up. Home to her is a place for rest and relaxation. She doesn't worry about tracking a little dirt into the house or eating in the living room. She's most comfortable with friends coming and going, newspapers strewn about. She likes to cook in the backyard on the grill or eat crabs over newspapers. She doesn't fret about a few dishes in the kitchen sink.

Mary's husband, Steve, believes his home

and its furnishings reflect his position in life. When he brings coworkers or friends into his home he expects everything to be in it's place, expects to feed them gourmet food, preferably at small dinner parties, and serves the best wine. His idea of fun is an opera, symphony, or the theater. He likes to discuss the latest literature.

Steve believes Mary's way of living shows she lacks consideration for her belongings, shows she doesn't care about his standing in the community, and lacks a deep meaning in her life. Initially Steve thought Mary was cute and fun to be around, now he sees her as a slob. Why couldn't she see her need to change and be more adult?

Mary thinks Steve is rigid and doesn't even know how to share himself in an unguarded way. She thinks he should loosen up and have some fun. Why can't he learn to play? What she thought was an adult sense of propriety she now believes is snobbery. She believes he's more concerned with appearances and keeps others at a distance. She feels frustrated that he seems to live in ideas rather than being engaged in life. Mary resents Steve's interpretation of her behavior, resents Steve's belief that his way of life is better.

Sharon fell in love with a midshipman attending the Naval Academy. The ritual and ceremony of his life at the academy fascinated her. She thought the whole idea of the navy and the academy was glamorous. Sharon and Eric counted the days to their wedding, which was planned to take place in the Naval Academy Chapel the day after Eric's graduation. Their wedding and honeymoon lived up to the high expectations Sharon had had all of her life. She was on cloud nine.

As soon as they returned from their honeymoon everything changed. The navy ordered Eric to report to a naval air station in Florida for flight training. Moving to Florida didn't bother Sharon, but worrying everyday about whether her husband would return bothered her a great deal. She made some new friends with other pilot wives, but Sharon longed to turn to her family and childhood friends for support. And when Eric was ordered out to sea for his first of many six-month tours, Sharon couldn't stand the loneliness. What if Eric never returned? Sharon could barely cope with his absence. On his return, though, she was faced with yet another dilemma. Eric wanted Sharon to do everything his way. He related to Sharon as if she were one of his crew. By the third year of this pattern they lived out each year, Sharon decided navy life wasn't for her. The emotional stress was more than she could take. What would she do if Eric were killed? How can you raise children with their dad gone six of every twelve months? How can you handle the confusion of their roles depending on whether Eric was home or not? Sharon simply couldn't live that life.

Work and Level of Ambition

Is your partner's work hard physical labor? How much energy do they have at the end of a workday? At the end of the workweek? Are they so active and social at work that they crave quiet time at home to rest? Do they have to work a lot of overtime to earn the amount of money it takes to support themselves? Do they sit inside at a desk all week and want to spend the week-end outdoors playing? Do they feel most productive when they put in additional hours of work at home? Does their work create a need for them to rehash and ventilate at home about stressful work they do? Do they walk out the door and leave their work behind, ready to devote leisure time to play and rest? Do their career plans include climbing an organizational ladder demanding long hours and social activities that further their career?

As you've already seen, differences in educational ambition can get in the way of a great marriage. The type of work you and your partner do and your levels of career ambition also affect your relationship for better or worse.

Your social status and your identity in our society are often determined by your job. He's a policeman. She's a doctor. The kind of work you do affects your lifestyle, the amount of money you have, the time and energy you have for your marriage and family, where to live, how you want to spend your leisure time, and your need for education. Your level of ambition further impacts upon the same characteristics.

Even under the best circumstances the effects of the kind of work you do spills over into your personal life, negatively or positively. A person in a high stress job, such as an emergency medical doctor or a policeman, may come home at the end of the day emotionally frazzled.

Their partner who is emotionally connected to them feels the effects of this emotional overload. In fact, many groups of emergency personnel offer support groups to family members.

A trap that you can easily fall into is to give more weight to this characteristic, wanting someone who makes a lot of money or is famous, to the exclusion of matching on the other fifteen characteristics.

Balance between work, your family, friends, and the time it takes to be actively involved in your partner's life is a critical issue. We'll talk more about balance as part of effectiveness when we ask you to answer one of the five questions used to determine whether someone is right for you.

Jerry has a passion for sales. He's been working in a variety of sales positions since college graduation to perfect his sales ability. He's born for sales, believes in his product, and has risen steadily in his industry.

Attracted to Jerry's enthusiasm for life, Nancy married Jerry believing he'd settle down after marriage to a more sedate life style. Jerry had expressed just as much desire to have a family as Nancy. Once the family started she believed Jerry would naturally be home more often, putting work on the back burner. She believed he'd want to do work with a more predictable income. Her father had settled into a nine to five routine in his marriage to her mother, arranging his life however his wife wanted it arranged.

Nancy wasn't prepared for Jerry's resistance to change anything about his career and work style. He'd always worked these hours. Where in the world did she ever get the idea that he intended to modify his life for a family? He thought he'd be a much better father doing the kind of work he loved. He knew he'd be a better husband engaged in work he liked to do.

Jerry tried to get Nancy into counseling, but she only wanted what she wanted and wouldn't go. Facing the reality of Nancy's expectations and demands and living as honestly and straightforwardly as he always had, Jerry ended the marriage after three months.

Jerry isn't a workaholic. He loves his work and his play. He spends more time at work than many people because of the business he's in; he spends some weekends and holidays at work because that's when people buy cars. But he doesn't spend endless hours at work. This is a case of mismatched expectations of marriage exemplified by someone's work.

Workaholics exemplify another set of circumstances that interfere with marriage. Workaholics tend to avoid intimacy and conflict by limiting their hours at home. Workaholics are often more concerned with appearances and climbing the work ladder than being actively involved in their marriage partner's life.

To have a great marriage your prospective partner's career goals must blend easily with your idea of life.

Views on How to Handle and Spend Money

Money is power, and the one who controls the money intrinsically has a more powerful place in the relationship. In your marriage, money can mean equal power with equal influence or an imbalance of power.

In reality, money is just money, representing an exchange for energy. But unfortunately, most people attach more meanings to money. The meanings you attach to money influence how you earn, spend and save money. How you earn, spend, and save money impacts on your marriage. You and your partner have to be able to comfortably blend your ways of managing money to circumvent the power and control fallout caused by a difference in how you handle your money.

Many variations of many themes concerning the earning, spending, and saving of money play themselves over and over in marriages. How much income does your partner want to save and spend? How much money do they want to allocate for clothes, vacations, gifts, savings, etc.? What amount of money do they want to give away and to whom? What is the degree of risk they're willing to take with investments? What do they believe about saving for retirement? Who's going to manage the money in their marriage? Who pays the bills? How will they decide what and how to spend or save? Will one partner be financially dependent on the other? If one partner agrees to be financially dependent, what will be done to assure a balance of power and an equitable division of assets in the event of divorce? Who will spend money on the children? Will they pool their money in joint accounts or separate their money and divide the bills?

As we said, the way you handle money often represents other attributes about yourself and other meanings you attach to money. Three types of spenders are worth considering in depth while seeking a marital partner. If you run into a miser, someone who goes to the extreme of not spending money, please consider their behavior overall for stinginess. A lack of generosity can represent a closed heart, someone that withholds intimacy, affection, and love. At the other extreme, a spendthrift may be careless about living within any kind of budget, may be irresponsible about money as well as your marriage. Expensive gifts and special attention may be romantic and elevate your self-esteem, but at what expense? Do you want to deal with poor credit ratings or maybe even bankruptcy? The third type, someone who refuses to pool their income with yours and wants to separate the bills may seriously limit your ability to have any kind of intimacy in your marriage. Separate money can mean separate lives, different goals, and lack of trust.

Attention to similarities and differences about earning, spending, and saving money between you and your prospective marriage partner can save you from the conflict and heartache of marrying the wrong person.

Susan's childhood experiences with money impacted on her marriage. Her husband Joe was an engineer and quite bright and talented. Joe had difficulty fitting-in in organizational work situations, probably because he's so smart and creative. Not content with the status quo, he made job changes frequently, which was extremely unsettling to Susan. Every time Joe ended one job, he found something equally good or even better within a short period of time. Even so, Susan would come severely unglued. Susan's mother and father had divorced during her childhood. Her father paid his child support inconsistently and frequently paid late. Her mother dealt with this by sending Susan over to get money from her father. Being the go-between in such an emotionally loaded situation created high anxiety for her. The new money situation triggered the old anxiety. Susan and Joe fought about earning, spending, and saving money. The idea of running out of money not only frightened Susan, but it seemed to her as if Joe didn't even care about her security.

Ralph and Jean's marriage was riddled with conflict. These two had so many areas of mismatch that the simplest decisions and actions often provoked disagreement. Their relationship evolved into a huge power struggle over basic living rights. Even though Ralph was the primary breadwinner, Jean managed all of the money. Ralph liked sex often, the less the better for Jean. Jean used giving or withholding sex to get Ralph to do what she wanted. She often maligned Ralph to their daughter. Jean controlled any money spent on the children, which further decreased Ralph's credibility in their eyes.

In Carolyn's previous marriage she had a partner that believed his funds were limited. If he saw something he wanted, but it didn't fit into his normal budget, he'd forego its purchase. He said, "we can't afford that", many times. Carolyn approached the same situation by working an extra shift to earn whatever she needed to make the purchase. She never saw herself as not being able to afford something. She could always work more and earn more.

Many of us have parents from the generation that endured the big depression. We both have parents that have. Both our fathers restrict their spending as if the next big depression is just around the corner. Both our fathers use all kinds of manipulation and control to keep our mothers from spending money the way they would with no outside control. Both of our mothers have to buy some items discreetly, or face an interrogation about why they're trying to put themselves and our dads into the poor house. Both couples have eroded trust and love over the issue of spending and saving money.

Among other examples, Wes's mom had to defend herself and beg for mercy once when she bought a purse for a hundred dollars. She'd mentioned she bought a "wallet" instead of a purse and when Wes's dad saw the credit card bill he raised the roof. It wasn't until she brought out the 15-year-old purse she'd replaced and explained she meant she'd bought a purse not a wallet that he settled himself down and behaved reasonably. On another occasion she stumbled across a good deal on some outdoor furniture for their deck and bought it. She heard about that for days. When she began getting her own social security check, she opened her own checking account in which to have it deposited automatically. When Wes's dad found out her check went into her own account he went ballistic. But understanding why she would open her own account isn't difficult to understand. Even more assertively, another time, Wes's mom, made a real estate venture. After years of renting the property she decided to sell it as it had become too much work to manage. When they did their income tax and had to pay the capital gains tax on the sale Wes's dad complained and belittled her decision to try her hand at that kind of an investment. Wes's mom has learned that stashing away cash and buying the things she needs for cash saves her a lot of grief. Such disagreements about how to spend and save money erode trust and affection over time; such disagreements breed power struggles, deception, and resentment. Money disagreements are no-win situations.

Carolyn's mother never got a chance to learn how to handle money and was criticized constantly for how she handled the money she did get her hands on. Carolyn's father kept the amount of his paycheck a secret from her mother throughout his working life. He feared if she knew how much he earned she would spend all of it. When her mother brought up the idea of getting her own job and earning her own money, Carolyn's dad nixed the idea because, he said, it would raise their taxes to the next tax percentage. Like Wes's mother, Carolyn's mother went through all of her married years learning how to buy the things she wanted on the sly. When Carolyn's mother inherited her own money from her parents, Carolyn's dad wanted her to turn it over to him. Her mother resisted under heavy fire. After all, her dad reasoned, he'd shared his money with her...or had he? In the end, her mother turned some of the money over to her husband, but she also kept some of the money regardless of the ongoing verbal assault. Eventually, Carolyn's mother decided to invest some of her money in two ventures to try her hand at increasing her capital. Both ventures fizzled, so she heard about her stupidity for a very long time. There was even some discussion that she was incompetent to handle their financial affairs. But what would you expect from someone who'd never handled her own money before? She never had an opportunity to make smaller mistakes at a younger age. How could she learn to manage money unless she had a chance to manage some? Making the mistakes earlier in life might have prevented these investment mistakes from happening at a time in their life when they lived on a fixed income and couldn't afford to make up for a loss. Or, better yet, they could have benefited from the extra income from a good investment.

Can you imagine the kind of control and power games people have to play when they disagree about managing money?

Expectations of Marriage

Our agent once asked us, "Don't people expect too much from marriage?" Carolyn's immediate reply was, "People don't expect enough from their marriage."

When something happens that you don't like, like a bad marriage, you look around for the cause. It's easy to assign a cause that may not be true. When you can't produce a desired outcome by the behaviors you use over and over, often, you lower your expectations. Lowering your expectations for marriage becomes a self-fulfilling prophecy. You get what you expect. You get what you set your sights on. Marriages can be great, with a high level of mutual satisfaction. But you do have to set your sights on that target.

When you choose the wrong partner, no matter how skillful you become at relating to others, incompatibility limits satisfaction. Talking yourself out of what you want erodes the trust you have in yourself and leads to self-doubt, persistent disappointment and a sense of failure, powerlessness, and hopelessness. Talking yourself out of what you want gives away the real power you do have to get what you want.

One of the most common complaints of men after divorce is that they never got enough sex. Doomed to never feeling sexually satisfied, men turned that into believing that women don't like sex. But that isn't true. It's a myth. In a survey we did, more women than men said that sex was very important. So many women do like sex that a generalized assumption that women don't like sex is just plain wrong.

More than likely, the men with that complaint have married the wrong partner. Their sex drives don't match. Or they don't match on other important characteristics and the woman withdraws sex from lack of desire or out of anger because of their ongoing conflict or resentment. Or the women they pick fit their expectation and don't like sex for some reason or another. Or maybe the man doesn't know how to satisfy that particular woman, the woman fails to teach him what to do to satisfy her, and her perpetual dissatisfaction builds resentment and disinterest in sex.

The most important expectation about marriage is the level of intimacy you desire from your relationship with your mate. Does your mate want to be your best friend, your confidante? Do they want to spend as much time with you as possible, or do they want to split their time and confidences between other friends and you?

We're of the opinion that to have a great marriage you must have a high level of emotional safety; a great marriage offers the kind of safety to each other in which your deepest joys and fears can be shared. You'll achieve the best you can have when your mate is the one person you can trust with everything about yourself. Within a small window can be some variation that includes another close friend in whom you may confide. But that window is very small. Sharing confidences takes time and energy. If you split time and energy for intimacy between your mate and others you'll diminish the potential for intimacy in your marriage. A great marriage can only happen when the emotional environment is such that mutual disclosure of your real selves – intimacy – comes naturally.

Set your sights on the target you want, and select a partner with the same expectation for the level of intimacy that you want from your marriage.

What does your partner expect from their marriage? Do they want a traditional marriage where the husband earns the money and his wife stays home with the children? Do they want careers for both partners to prevail with or without children? Do they want to marry their best friend? Do they want their marriage to be at the center of their life? Or do they want to put their career first? Do they want to maintain other friendships with people that serve as their confidant? Do they want to spend their leisure time with you or with other friends? How much time do they want to spend alone with you?

Sam and Trisha are married and have two young children. They illustrate the dilemma of many young, modern families. Like most young men and women these days, Sam and Trisha believe in the value of women in the workplace. Both of them believed they wanted Trisha to be a working mother. When Trisha had her first child she began to do work for her company at home. During the years of raising her two children while working at home she came to love being at home. Both children are now in school full time and it's time for Trisha to return to the workplace. But she doesn't want to go. She wants to have another child and stay at home. Sam wants her added income and wants her to return to work. Someone is going to lose in this situation.

John and Rosemary have lived together for seven years. Rosemary wants to get married and have all of the status and recognition of marriage. John refuses to divorce his wife because his father wouldn't approve, he doesn't want his wife to drag him through anticipated mudslinging, and he doesn't want to alienate his children. Besides, he loves Rosemary. He never wants to be with anyone else except Rosemary. He just doesn't understand why Rosemary is so upset. Unfortunately, every time Rosemary tries to talk herself out of marriage and into accepting things as they are, she fills with anguish and resentment. Her love and affection for John is buried under so much hostility that we doubt they'll ever recapture their love, even if John decides to marry her eventually. Rosemary values marriage deeply which makes talking herself out of believing in marriage impossible. She feels even worse because John doesn't value marriage enough to marry her. No amount of justification or rationalization will change her belief in and desire for marriage.

Differentiate your expectation of marriage from the expectations of others. Then choose a partner that wants the same that you want from your marriage.

Physical Characteristics Attractive to You

Certain types of bodies are more attractive to you than others. What physique does your partner like? Is there any characteristic that really turns him or her on? Does he or she like blondes, brunettes, or redheads? What style of clothes do they like?

When you pick a partner based solely on being attracted you make a big mistake. On the other hand, if you marry someone that matches you in other ways without an attraction to them physically, you make a big mistake, too. Over time, conflict in most areas of your life erodes any physical attraction that was there at the beginning. Over time, matching well in all the other differences that make a difference can lead to more physical attraction.

Stan was immediately attracted to Karen. He loved her body and the way she dressed. Drawn to her because of her sensuality and flirtation, he pursued a serious relationship. Even though Karen's dress and behavior led him to believe Karen was sensual and sexy, Stan couldn't get Karen to have sex very often. Stan believed Karen was holding out for marriage. So Stan married Karen. Only Karen's desire for sex never increased. She confused Stan because of her sexy style, but lack of desire for sex. Not only was Karen's behavior misleading about her desire for sex, but it turned out they had little compatibility for any of the other important characteristics. Their marriage became a nightmare of conflict and dissatisfaction because their marriage was based entirely on physical attraction.

Elaine was five feet nine inches tall. But she liked short men. Her parents and friends nagged Elaine to date taller men. So she tried it. She tried to build her appreciation for taller men, and even talked herself into marrying Dave who was six-three. Dave had many good qualities, she trusted him, she liked him; they had much in common. Even though Elaine admired and liked Dave, her feelings never grew into electricity. She wondered if this low-key day-to-day survival could sustain their marriage. One day Vic came along. Elaine had never been so attracted to anyone. And she had even more in common with Vic than she did with Dave. She began an affair. Elaine had sold out to someone else's idea of how her partner should look. But now she had a serious dilemma. Should she stay married to someone she likes as a friend, but with whom she feels trapped and limited. Or should she face the truth and divorce Dave in order to realize her dream of a great marriage. Vic not only energized Elaine, but he felt the same, and they had a high level of compatibility in every other characteristic.

Elaine obsessed about these two relationships and what she should do. The question was, should she sell out again to what everyone else thought she should do and stay with Dave? Or should she listen to herself and go for a great marriage? What would you do?

To facilitate Elaine's decision, Carolyn reflected to Elaine that coming to therapy for most people is difficult. It's so difficult that most people put it off until life or a crisis become unbearable. Coming into therapy signifies a problem that is deeply serious. Elaine should listen to herself acting on something very important. She needs to trust herself. She may not understand why this is happening, but the fact that it is and the intensity of her feelings suggests something important. Someone's height may seem a trite reason to divorce, but in this case, the chemistry and attraction to Vic adds an element to Elaine's life that energizes her to contribute her best to the world.

Something else to consider is that staying in her marriage traps Dave into a mediocre marriage. He feels hurt. A divorce from Elaine will cause distress and grief. But what could Dave have for himself if he were to find the right partner? Staying with Dave may seem the loving thing to do, but is it really? Acting in a loving way toward Dave means allowing the kind of freedom that facilitates his being all he can be. Sometimes causing pain for the moment is the most loving thing someone can do for another person. Doesn't loving behavior want the best for the other person? Isn't loving behavior usually honestly being who you are? Do you stop and think that sometimes protecting another person from emotional pain actually says you don't think them capable of handling a difficult situation? Isn't that a put down? Do you stop and think that you're really protecting yourself from criticism – from disapproval? Loving behavior is that that promotes stretching yourself and growth.

While Carolyn doesn't tell others what to do, she doesn't hesitate to give someone her opinion, along with leading the patient through a serious of questions designed to illustrate the issues and designed to evoke the kind of thinking that will help to resolve a problem. She makes sure the patient has understood all of the options available and then she offers her own opinion, knowing that, ultimately, people must decide – think for themselves. In this case, Carolyn believed both Dave and Elaine would be better off ending their marriage. Both should go for great, finding the right partner for a great marriage.

Elaine's first attempt to resolve her dilemma in therapy ended with her decision to stay in her marriage. But within a year she was back in therapy. Dave had begun to question their staying together by now and Elaine was back due to serious emotional turmoil. She loves Vic. She wants to be with Vic. But she wants to do what's right. She's confused about sacrifice and duty and commitment. Only this time, Dave wants out. He's begun to sense what finding the right partner could give to him.

The second time around, they decided to divorce. After a period of grief and emotional work in therapy to understand and resolve her guilt, Elaine and Vic were married. A year later, Dave found the right partner and he's remarried and says he has a great marriage. Both couples are planning families.

He Said

I like brunettes or redheads with pale skin. Something about the contrast between dark hair color and skin really turns me on. I'm also most attracted to women that take good care of themselves, staying fit and healthy. When a woman considers herself worth taking good care of she attracts men. Other physical characteristics don't matter too much. Physical characteristics would never be the only thing on which I base picking a partner, but when we match on other characteristics, I wouldn't even consider marrying someone I didn't consider attractive.

We're not speaking of Mr. or Mrs. America beauty here. Glamorous beauty isn't attractive very long if other characteristics about the person aren't attractive. We're speaking of the kind of inner beauty that a mature and confident person radiates when they take care of themselves and take care to present an attractive package to others.

You are the only one that can decide if a partner is attractive to you.

Religious Beliefs and Practices

How many times have you heard someone say not to discuss religion in social situations? Religious beliefs and practices are so personal and varied that opinions can easily spark conflict. But please don't apply that rule to the selection of a marriage partner. You must know what part religious beliefs and practices play in your mate's life. Your religious beliefs and practices determine the way you live your life; they determine your values.

Just as differences in political beliefs, differences in religious/spiritual beliefs and practices undermine emotional safety, respect, and acceptance.

As you look at what part religion plays in a potential mate's life and whether what they believe and do matches you well, determine their spiritual beliefs – what they believe – along with how they practice what they believe – religious ceremony. Does the basic premise of their

beliefs blend with what you believe? Is the way
they practice their beliefs compatible with the
way you practice your beliefs? How do they
believe children should be raised in regard to
spiritual beliefs? Will the blend of your spiritual beliefs and religious practices contribute to
the healthy function of your marriage? How will
the celebration of various holidays be affected
by the blend of your religious beliefs and practices? How will interaction with your extended
families be affected by the blend of your religious beliefs and practices?

Earl and Connie ran into marital trouble
when Earl shamed Connie about not attending
church. While dating, attending church wasn't
discussed. Connie went to church with Earl's
family when visiting a few times; Earl hadn't
mentioned attending church while visiting
Connie's family. Once married things changed.
Earl's family started putting pressure on them
to attend church. When Connie became pregnant the pressure intensified. Earl had been
raised to believe that attending church was the
way to practice your belief in God. Earl's mother put a lot of pressure on him to insist that
Connie go to church every Sunday. But Connie
had long since decided that church was not for
her. Her experiences had led her to lead her life
in what she believed was a conscientious effort
to practice spiritual teachings. To Connie, any
place could be a church. She particularly felt
spiritually at peace while hiking or gardening or
feeding the birds. She felt fine about the way
she practiced her beliefs.

But Earl and his family couldn't buy such

a thing. If you don't go to church you don't have religion. They put heavy stock in church activities. Nothing Connie could say reassured them of her spiritual beliefs. They simply couldn't tolerate this difference in attitude about religion. And what would happen to the children if they weren't taught to attend church each week?

Both Earl and Connie have a right to their beliefs. Religious and spiritual practices are personal expressions of your values. The only way to win is to match yourself with someone who's religious and spiritual expression closely resembles your own. Earl and Connie couldn't overcome their differences. Particularly, because Earl's family demanded his ongoing, undying loyalty in the matter. Earl and Connie divorced inside of a year after their child was born. Their irreconcilable differences about religious practice, the interference of Earl's family in the setting of his and Connie's own traditions and practices, caused a rift in their marriage that they couldn't repair. The power struggles about how to raise their child continue to this day, several years after their divorce. Often caught between her parents' wishes, their child often feels guilty and disloyal when she finds she can never satisfy anyone.

Political Beliefs and Practices

How many times have you heard someone say not to discuss politics at social gatherings? If you think political beliefs are divisive in social relationships, you should see how divisive political beliefs can be in a marriage. Politics is another area that reflects personal values. Differences easily spark conflict. Depersonalizing a conflict of political beliefs is difficult because your political beliefs and practices fit what you believe about life. Cooperating and getting along by tolerating differences in political beliefs in a marriage can only compromise what you believe, draining energy from your activities. If you feel strongly about something and your mate feels differently, you lose respect and emotional connection. How can you be married to someone who votes for someone you despise?

What are your partner's political beliefs and practices? What part do your partner's politics play in his or her life? How do their political beliefs reflect their values? What role do they believe the government should play in their life? Do they believe in more or less government? Do they think taxes are too high, too low, or just about right? What kind of beliefs do they have that would fit with your beliefs?

In Carolyn's first marriage she submitted to her husband, Steve, who dominated. In most issues what he wanted was what happened. Carolyn rarely spoke of her views and opinions about any issue. She never discussed politics because what she believed was different from her husband and his family.

The first issue to surface regarding their political beliefs was whether or not Steve would go to Vietnam. No small issue. Fortunately, their marriage and birth of their first child relieved Steve from having to go to war. He wouldn't have gone anyway, he figured. He'd move to Canada first. Carolyn didn't like the Vietnam War, but believed that if it was going to be fought it should be fought to win. She couldn't bear the idea of her new husband going off to war, but believed in her country and believed her husband should accept his responsibility as a citizen.

Other issues surfaced over time. Taxes and a poor economy reinforced Carolyn's ideas about the strength of a free market. Her husband believed in more government programs. Carolyn believed helping others was best achieved through teaching them how to take care of themselves, not doing for the other person. That belief influenced how they each believed children should be raised. Carolyn believed her job as a parent was to teach her children how to think for themselves and take care of themselves. Steve tended to do things for his sons and take care of them.

Carolyn's beliefs in helping others influenced her to work with emotionally disturbed kids in an inner city. For twelve years, she drove into the city, often working 16 hours a day with the kids and their families, teaching them how to take control of their lives. Steve and his family, who professed to care compassionately about helping the disadvantaged (through government programs and taxes) couldn't fathom her working in such a dangerous environment.

More recently, 13 years after their parents' divorce, two of Carolyn's sons think she's become extreme in her political thinking (even though they basically believe as she does). In relation to her never having opened her mouth during their early years to express her opinion, she now freely articulates what she believes. Carolyn's ideas haven't changed at all, but she is more assertive and speaks openly about her beliefs.

You might be tempted to say that when two parents have differing political beliefs the children get a broader view from which to base their own political beliefs. Unfortunately, that's not what happens. What it feels like to the children is that they have to choose between loyalty to each of their parents. Role modeling diverse beliefs from the general human audience broadens the experience for children, offering them an opportunity to think through the issues from many angles. Role modeling from your parents provides a more solid sense of security if they have similar beliefs and practices. Children grow best when their parents are united and strong in their beliefs, while maintaining a broad exposure for their children, to the world at large.

Children – having them and raising them

After deciding on whether you want to have children and how many, as parents, you need to agree on your basic philosophy of how to raise children. Does your partner want children? How many children do they want? What do they believe is effective discipline for children? How structured do they believe your children's lives should be? Do they want to have stepchildren or more children with a new mate? What do they believe about mothers working? What do they believe about the roles of parents? How would they like to distribute the household workload associated with running a home with children? Is their lifestyle compatible with the needs of children? Is their income adequate for the number of children they want? Is their energy level adequate for the number of children they want?

Children take concerted effort and attention to raise. When their mother and father have the same ideas about marriage and parenting, raising their children is much easier than with a perpetual tug of war going on. When their parents are free of the distractions of making their own relationship work, they're free to attend to their children. When their parents have high regard and admiration for each other much less confusion about life is created for the children. Parents are free to support one another when they agree on their way of life. Children will have plenty of opportunity to observe and decide for themselves about different ways of living without it coming from their parents. Having a high level of compatibility on these 16 differences models selecting the right marriage partner for their children.

First, know what you believe in regard to having and raising children, and then match yourself to someone with compatible ideas and behaviors.

Alan and Kathy battle constantly about how to reward and punish their children. They don't agree on much of anything in regard to raising their children. In general, Kathy believes structure offers children predictability and knowledge about how to organize their daily routines. Alan thinks Kathy interferes too much in their lives. He says children should make their own decisions and learn from their mistakes. Kathy would prefer they never made mistakes.

Unfortunately, the children have learned to play their parents off against each other. As long as Alan and Kathy are distracted by their disagreement on how to handle the children, the children don't have to take responsibility for their behavior. Everyone's too busy to notice. The children have learned to play people off against each other no matter where they are, at a neighbor's house, at school, in the community. This family's days are filled with conflict and stress. Every member is exhausted from the turmoil.

In Diane's and Mickey's family the children accept responsibility for their behavior and eagerly seek added responsibility as they mature. None of the children are geniuses, but all four of them get average to above average grades in school. Their relationships with peers are filled with fun and pleasure. The children are good at problem solving.

What's makes the difference? Diane and Mickey agree on the role of parents with children. Their ideas about life and raising children have a high level of compatibility. Because of their compatibility they can support one another whenever the circumstances warrant support. The key is that they match each other.

Life Stage

What tasks are your partner busy with in their life? Are they still in school, yet to begin a career? Maybe they've been out of school and have settled into their first job. Are they divorced with children in elementary, middle or high school? Are they looking for a new mate just short of their own retirement from the work force? Are they putting young adult children through college? The tasks that fill your life at the moment create a stage in your life.

It's much easier to create a great marriage when partners are at the same stage in life. At times slight differences will work, but even slight differences at certain stages can make life difficult. Differences in age can place you in different life stages, but doesn't necessarily. We're the same age, but at different stages in raising our children. Carolyn's children are finished with college, into their careers, and married. Wes's children are 23 and 17. None of our children live in our household. This particular difference doesn't make much difference. It does drag out paying college bills longer for Carolyn, but life in general is the same for both of us.

Andy and Janice have a little bit of difficulty because Andy's just retired and Janice has five years to go before she can even think about retirement. Andy gets to name his daily routine, but Janice has to get up and go to work and turn the light out at a decent hour. Andy's free to go fishing and travel; Janice's job restricts what they can do together.

Phil is 29 and single. He's in love with Carrie who is the young, 30-year-old mother of three. Phil wants to get married, but Carrie doesn't want to have anymore children. Phil wants a big family and several of his own children.

Arlene and Justin want to get married, but Arlene has two teenage sons and a teenage girl. None of the children like the idea of Justin living with their mom, let alone telling them what to do. Trying to survive with the power struggles and leaps to independence with a new character in the play usually makes circumstances worse rather than better; it is in this case. Arlene longs to return to a peaceful household without all of the conflict and negotiation. She loves Justin, she loves her children, and she loves her former active, but peaceful life. Will they live through the chaos?

Choose a mate that matches the life stage in which you find yourself.

Leisure Interests

A great marriage depends on active participation in your partner's life.

Add up the number of hours you work, the time you spend commuting, sleeping, learning new skills, and doing the work required to run your home and raise your children and you'll see that not many hours remain for relaxation and fun. If you spend your leisure time apart from your partner you'll have precious little time together. Intimacy depends on attachment and bonding – on building a history together. If you don't spend time together you won't reinforce your bond.

Relaxation and fun balance the work of life, recharge your batteries, relieve stress, and contribute to mental and physical health. Relaxation and fun together fortify the bond between marriage partners. Associating your spouse with the fun and relaxation in your life adds to your love and affection for one another.

Leisure interests encompass all sorts of active and passive entertainment like television, movies, plays, dancing, listening to music, bird watching, travel, clubs in the community, church activities, reading. Watching or participating in sports are other activities people spend their leisure time doing. Just about anything can be done for fun.

What's fun for one person can be work for another person. What does your partner like to do with their leisure time? What kinds of activities contribute to their well being? What would they like to be able to do with you during leisure time?

Life can be hard work. First, learn to balance your own work life with fun. Then select a partner that enjoys the same kind of activities.

Liz and Herb have been married eighteen years and have two school age children. They've had a moderately comfortable life. They grew up together and fell into marriage after high school. Both work and participate in community activities. Both coach and organize little league activities for young people in their town. Unfortunately, they never do any of these activities together. They run into each other once in a while at home, but are so caught up in racing to beat the schedule and fit so many commitments into the day, they rarely see each other. By the end of the day they're exhausted and have no time left except to sleep. Sex is rare. Add to this the fact that Liz feels that her first loyalty is to her mother who has been sick almost all of Liz's life. Liz and Herb are well thought of in their community. Their children are high achievers in their busy lives. The community depends on them to help out as much as possible.

One day Herb came home and asked for a divorce. Liz couldn't imagine why. Haven't they all been happy in their busy lives? Most ironic was that, Liz didn't even really care. Surprised that she had so little feeling one way or the other about Herb's request, she said okay. Liz even thought Herb's falling in love with his old high school sweetheart was okay if that's what he wanted. After eighteen years of marriage everyone, including Liz and Herb, felt surprised at the seemingly little sadness and grief over the dissolution of their marriage. They hadn't realized they'd stopped loving each other many years before.

Avoid being caught by surprise. Avoid growing apart. Avoid putting your own companionship on the bottom of the list. Recognize the vital importance of active participation in your partner's life. Remember the value of a great marriage. Choose a marriage partner that balances work with play. Select a mate that shares a variety of leisure interests with you.

Energy Levels

People have different energy levels. Your energy level regulates your activity through each day and from day to day. Your energy level fluctuates throughout the day and night. Different people have more or less energy at different times of the day.

Is your mate someone with a high, moderate, or low energy level? What time of the day are they most physically energetic? When are they least physically energetic? When are they mentally sharp? When is their thinking the most sluggish? Do they jump out of the bed bright and early, eager to start the day? Or would they rather sleep late? Do they start to unwind toward late afternoon and go to bed by eleven? Or do they just get going for the day late morning or early afternoon, only to feel at their best as the sun goes down? Do they like to hike or ride a bike to see the sights, or would they rather ride in their car?

Julie's first husband, Dwight, never sits down. Sitting bores him. He sits at a desk all week and during his time off he wants to get out and do something. Julie is on her feet all day at work. Her job takes a lot of physical and mental energy. On her days off from work she wants to stay home and take it easy.

To cope with their difference in energy level they split their two-day weekend. Julie stays home and putters around the house on Saturday and Dwight spends the day working on his boat or his car. They spend Sunday together, but since Dwight can't sit still they usually go out. Julie wishes they could stay home together for a whole day at a time once in a while. But her choice is to spend most of her time away from Dwight or to go along with his desire for activity. Both choices are a losing proposition for Julie. It isn't that Dwight doesn't want to give Julie what she wants, he'd like to. But he can't change his energy level. Julie's chronic disappointment and feeling tired at the beginning of every week wears on her feelings for Dwight. Irritable most of the time, her tiredness wears on all of her interactions.

Donna and Vince have many common interests. They both enjoy movies, golf, entertaining friends and family at home, and their six children. Eating new food in new restaurants is an adventure. In measuring their compatibility they score relatively high. Unfortunately, Vince is a morning person and Donna is a night person. Donna and Vince struggle to find times of the day where they both have the energy to do what they like to do. They often end up going their separate ways because their energy levels are high and low at different times of the day. Their sex lives suffer because one is just getting started after dinner and wants to spend the evening working or reading or going to a movie. But Vince is asleep by nine or ten each night. He can't stay awake. They tried sex in the morning so Donna can stay in bed longer, but Vince feels like he's wasting half of the day.

This couple has so much positive reinforcement going for them in terms of their compatibility on our 16 characteristics that it balances the negative. But they don't get to spend as much time with each other as they'd like. Their temporary solution to this problem is muddling from day-to-day. They take time off from work to be together, spending that time reinforcing their affection and bond by doing fun activities together. But that time is limited. Their long-term solution is their goal to retire early, by the age of sixty, so they can blend their schedules for more time together. Under their circumstance they'll probably not suffer the long-term consequences of living separate lives – growing apart. This is their second marriage, they married about ten years ago, and they only have four years until they retire. And, they've taken interim measures to balance this negative drain on their relationship.

Your overall energy level and the rhythm of your energy level contribute positively to or tax your relationship. Give your marriage a boost by choosing a partner whose energy level matches yours. If you're a morning person, marry a morning person; if you're a night person, marry a night person.

It Should Have Been a Storybook Romance...

All the money in the world couldn't save Prince Charles and Princess Diana. Consider their marriage as an example of mismatched mates. Their marriage ended in divorce after two children; and they were often bitterly unhappy before their separation. The ultimate blow,

Diana's young and untimely death, was an indirect result of her unhappy marriage. Yet, their marriage should have been a storybook romance. Why did it fail? Why did Diana marry Prince Charles? He was handsome, rich, powerful, and famous. He romanced her. She believed he loved her. How could she go to her family and tell them that she had turned down such an offer? She couldn't, so she married him. Why did Charles marry Princess Diana? She was 18 years old. A beautiful woman. At age 31, he was getting a lot of pressure from the Queen of England to stop playing the field, settle down and have an heir to the throne. Charles had a very limited pool of women from which to select. Even if many women would have liked to marry Charles, and he them, his parents limited his choices. There are few women they would accept as the future Queen of England. Why did their marriage fail? Simply, they weren't good friends before they got married, and they had too many differences to overcome.

Everything you have in common with your marriage partner contributes to an effortless compatibility that frees your time and energy to engage in and enjoy life, to master the challenges of life. Such natural compatibility fuels respect, affection, and loving behaviors between you and your partner. Once you've matured and mastered competence at tasks of daily living, matching on these 16 differences that make a difference is the major key to a great marriage.

Part III

The Search

How and Where to Find Your Perfect Partner

6

Market Yourself

Be Attractive to Yourself First, Dress For Success, Go For Volume, Look in the Right Places

Romantic accidents rarely cause great marriages. So here we are, recommending a practical, step-by-step process for something we've all been taught should be romantic. And, somehow, romance got tangled up with accidental. But who says? Why could romantic only happen from an accident? Is such a notion really true?

No. Great marriages rarely happen from romantic accidents. It is much more difficult than you think to find someone who matches you closely. Mathematically, the number of ways that you can match on the 16 differences that make a difference is 65,536. Randomly pick two people from anywhere in the world and you only have 1 chance in 65,536 that they will match exactly. In practical terms the odds are not quite that high because you tend to be around people who live near you and who are similar to you culturally. But the odds are still very high. If you were in a room with 1,000 people of the opposite sex who were the same age, you'd be lucky to find five who matched you exactly. You'd have to date 200 hundred people to have a reasonable chance of finding one who matched.

With these kinds of odds, if you rely on romantic accidents, as so many before you have, you'll do as they do and end up as they do – in bad marriages or marriages of convenience. Look for your perfect partner on purpose – with intention – and dramatically improve your chance to find the great marriage you want.

Our finding each other was no accident. We found each other in the practical way we describe to you here. Our experience gave us an exhilarating, worry free, arena in which to fall in love. The romance had never been so good. You know why? It was because we were so certain about each other. We just knew we belonged together. No mystery, no guessing, no educated risks. The fear and emotional roller coaster were non-existent. Just fun, and joy, and happiness. The result of falling in love this way is stunning.

Others criticized that we didn't know what we were getting into. We hadn't known each other long enough. They waited for us to wake up as they or others they knew had, lonely, frightened, and miserable. You know what? It didn't and won't happen. A few years later we feel more certain of each other and ourselves than ever. You want to talk about romance? Romance is a constant, daily quality of our love and of our lives.

Carolyn's experience with patients finding perfect partners has deepened our belief that this approach works well. Watching her patients undergo a complete change in attitude and behavior about relationships, love, and marriage after getting their heads straight proved that the most beneficial work you can do about relationships is on yourself and your approach.

Market Yourself

On the dating scene, marketing yourself is about developing your personal power. More personal power means more choices and more freedom. The ideas that good marketing and sales people have created can help you deal with fierce competition in the dating marketplace. Marketing can help you prepare for and deal with dating's disadvantages – it can be hard work, emotionally bruising, and expensive in time, money, and energy. Many people in the dating marketplace are bitter and hostile because they've been taken advantage of so many times. Marketing yourself will help you overcome these barriers by making you so attractive that even the jaded people will be interested in you. And truth in advertising applies.

In the dating marketplace you are both a buyer and a seller. You've got to let others – in large numbers – know you're available. And when you find someone that interests you, you have to sell yourself – convince the other person that they should go on a date with you and eventually marry you.

The first time Wes used the words "sell yourself" Carolyn cringed. She said, "we can't tell women to sell themselves." We bantered back and forth a little with Carolyn finally convincing Wes that just using those words could undermine our message. However, selling yourself is involved in the process of marrying your perfect partner. So the best way around this obstacle of what to call the process is to begin right here to change your mind and attitude about the words "sell yourself". We are not talking about selling your body. We are talking about assuring a prospective perfect partner that you are what he or she says they want, if it's really true.

Your marketing plan:
- Be attractive to yourself first – build your self- esteem.
- Dress for success – build your self-confidence.
- Go for volume – meet and date as many people as you can – successful dating builds self-confidence.
- Look in the right places.

-Honesty and integrity pay off – disclose
the real you.
-Be attractive to yourself first.

Have you ever noticed how much easier it
is to believe a sales person that believes in their
product? You are about to take yourself into the
dating marketplace to look for your perfect partner. Nothing conveys whom you are to a
prospective partner better than how you feel
about yourself and the way that shows itself in
your activity. One of the primary tasks of
preparing yourself to find the right partner is to
know and like yourself first. We've talked to you
extensively about that and it was in preparation
of your taking yourself into the world as you
really are. You are your product. And the dating
marketplace is where you present yourself to
potential partners. Look purposefully for the
partner you want.

The way you look and live must reflect the
real you. Despite the advice offered in popular
books like The Rules, which urge women to
play hard to get, tricks and manipulation always
backfire. How do you have intimacy when
you've established your relationship on distance and mystery? How can you find out if you
match if you keep your distance? How do you
find your perfect partner when you pretend
you're not looking?

Your reputation with yourself – what you
think of the way you think and act – is the most
important gauge you have for yourself. No other
opinion matters more. Modest belief in your
product (not grandiosity or arrogance and a

sense of entitlement, but real confidence) will sell you to the right person faster than any scheme or head game and with a far greater chance of a good match than any other thing you can do. You be the judge first.

People that feel attractive are healthy and fit and don't make excuses about how others should like them "for themselves". They stand up straight and make eye contact. They have energy to engage in life and they do engage in life.

Realize that asking others to like you for yourself if you are unhealthy, unfit, and your appearance outdated will attract people that don't care about health and fitness. What will they be like? Will they take care of themselves? Will they count your needs as worthy of time and energy, if you don't?

Attractive people update their look periodically. They keep their bodies and clothes clean and in good repair because it matters.

Attractive people have good manners. They respect social conventions in social places. If you need to learn about manners and social conventions, read a book or two about manners and etiquette. You don't have to be stuffy to be polite. Attractive people respect themselves and others. Their basic sense of respect is demonstrated in what they think and do. Manners apply equally to every class and situation except maybe some rescue or law-and-order circumstances.

Downplaying yourself, or even worse, self-depreciation and self-effacing behavior may be politically correct and demure behavior for women, but what does it say about you? Is it a copout so not too many demands will be made on you to participate in contributing to the world? Is it just an act with the expectation that someone will talk you out of feeling that way so you can win admiration and praise to bolster sagging self-esteem or a game you play to be praised? Or do you really mean you're worth less? Does it say you'll always be available to meet their needs because you don't have to spend any time on yourself? What does that behavior say about a man? Does it say he's passive and doesn't have a backbone? Either way, self-depreciation and self-effacement will attract partners that feel more comfortable, in control when their partner makes no demands. They make no demands even for meeting their most basic needs. That kind of partner feels that any expectation you may have that they will meet your needs is excessively demanding.

Katie, 25 years old, is an example of a young woman that demonstrated daily in multiple ways that she lacked self-confidence and sought approval from others rather than from herself. When she came to therapy, she'd had a string of relationships with young men that related to her by manipulation and control. Within weeks of the beginnings of their relationship the young men began showing up late, consistently, for dates. They rarely called ahead and sometimes didn't show up at all. If Katie asked about their behavior, these young men resorted to demeaning her and name-calling to discredit Katie's desire for respect. An even bigger problem was that Katie rarely asked about their behavior and never set reasonable limits like refusing to date them unless they showed up on time for dates. Katie's behavior said loud and clear that she would take less than respectful, mature behavior.

How did Katie tell others to treat her that way? The way you behave tells others how to treat you. Some people would never take advantage of someone who has low self-esteem by treating them with disrespect even at their invitation, but many would.

Are you surprised to learn that how Katie acted contributed to how others treated her? Katie exhibited low feelings about herself – which had everything to do with her behavior – in the manner in which she groomed and dressed herself. Her appearance described chapters about who she was before a single word ever came out of her mouth. She was overweight and wore loose clothes. She wore dark colors all of the time. Her hair went unwashed for several days. Her hairstyle was out-dated. She didn't wear any cosmetics and didn't take care of her skin.

Katie said she felt good about herself, but her behavior didn't match what she said.
Katie attracted men who wanted to control and manipulate because they could tell they could get away with that kind of behavior. She didn't attract respectful men because she didn't demonstrate respect for herself.

The way you act influences how others treat you.

When Carolyn asked Katie to think about what her appearance said about herself, Katie resisted the idea that appearance matters for weeks. She'd say things like "people should like me for who I am, not how I dress or fix my hair"; or "I don't care about nice clothes; I'm much more interested in my work". Okay, fine. Then all you'll attract are men that are willing to accept someone more interested in their work than themselves and men that don't care whether others like you because it makes you more available to them. They won't have to share.

As Katie worked through her feelings about herself and learned about who she really is, gradually, she began to treat herself differently. Small changes in her daily behavior included a new haircut, some new clothes, a small amount of makeup, and skin care. She did her nails. She began to care about her health. She was tired of having colds all of the time. She read about what she could do to improve her health and ability to fight colds. She changed her diet and began to exercise. Her skin cleared up. Her clothes included a variety of colors that were becoming to her.

She liked feeling healthy, strong, and energetic. She said she liked feeling womanly. She stood up straight and looked people in the eye. She liked the new kinds of people that befriended her. Her new friends were more willing to give and take rather than expecting to receive all of the time. Friends that expected her to give all of the time stopped seeing her because they didn't like "the new and selfish" Katie. She spent more time having fun than catering to others. She liked the new daily successes she was having in her life. Most of all, she stopped worrying about attracting everyone and winning praise from others. She became more aware that some peoples' measures don't work for her. She started setting her own goals and achieving them.

And she looked great. No burning beauty, but that inner glow that you've read about became part of her life. Her eyes sparkled and she smiled from inside. She felt relaxed and peaceful and it showed. And people responded positively, which reinforced how good she felt about herself. Her confidence grew.

Katie started to attract the kind of men that met the criteria of our five crucial questions. She dated several that met some of the criteria, but the first few didn't meet them all. She realized she was getting closer to her perfect partner. It wasn't long before she met Jim. And Katie could answer all five of the questions (Chapter 8) affirmatively.

The kind of people that meet the criteria of the five questions – the questions that tell you whether someone has what it takes to be your perfect partner – do care about how they and others take care of themselves and how they dress. It is a fact. No amount of wishful thinking and lowered expectations will ever attract someone who is solidly together himself or herself. It matters. Demonstrate that you care about yourself.

Translate your inner sense of worth into your appearance and behavior.

Dress for Success

There's an old saying that "clothes make the man," that you become what you seem to be. Your self-image and the way you dress are closely connected. You can change the way you see yourself by changing the way you dress. When you change the way you dress, you change how other people see and react to you. When you dress better, and other people reflect more positively on you, you see yourself more positively.

In 1975, John T. Molloy wrote a book called Dress For Success which was the result of extensive studies about how attire affects peoples' careers. The major points of his book are:

-Other's perceptions of how you look are
likely to be different from your
perception of how you look.
-Other's perceptions of how you look have
a stronger influence on how they see
you than you think.

Molloy illustrates these points repeatedly, but one of the best examples concerns the length of hair of a group of young male lawyers. All thought their hairstyles were modest. Molloy didn't agree, so he had drawings made of just their hairstyles and had them show these drawings to senior partners in their law firm. The senior partners all made negative comments about these hairstyles. Molloy says, "What you think about your hair length and style is totally irrelevant; what society thinks is largely irrelevant too. What matters are the opinions of those men who are in positions to make judgments about you that will either help or hurt."

Now, we don't agree that what you think about your hair style is totally irrelevant, because we believe that, in looking for a long-term partner, it's important to reveal your real self. But there's a powerful lesson here and that is:

You're never going to find the right partner if you can't get a date with someone who'd make a good long-term partner for you.

-How you dress and how you look is going
  to have a big impact on whether you
  can get a date with someone that
  interests you.
-If you don't think that looking good is
  important, you are underestimating its
  importance.

The best strategy is to dress as well as or slightly better than the best dressed people in the marketplace where you're looking for a partner.

We have both experienced decisions about how to dress and how it impacted on whom we attracted.

Wes remembers that it occurred to him that he should have new clothes for his new single, starting to date again, status. Reflecting the frugality he'd learned as a child, he initially bought clothes that were nice, but discounted.

After limited success in getting dates, he realized that he needed to improve his appearance. He'd begun feeling better about himself, even feeling excited that there was someone out there that would love him, and he reflected that in his desire for nice clothes. So he went shopping again.

He said that he realized that finding the right marriage partner was the most important thing in his life and that it meant putting all of his resources into the effort to find the right person. That included nice clothes. So he bought the nicest clothes he could buy and live within his income. It made a difference. Wes remembers that he started getting more and better dates immediately.

Carolyn remembers realizing one day that many people commented on how tired or well she looked and their comments didn't always coincide with the way she felt. She began to wonder what made the difference. It dawned on her that the colors she wore influenced how others reacted to her and how they perceived her. Carolyn headed for the bookstore (Carolyn's stepdaughter once commented that Carolyn had a book for everything). At the bookstore she found the book she wanted: <u>Color Me Beautiful</u>. In the back of her mind she'd remembered hearing about the system that this author had devised for helping people wear the colors most becoming to them based on their skin tone.

According to the system in <u>Color Me Beautiful</u>, Carolyn had been wearing many of the wrong colors for her skin.

Changing the colors in her wardrobe made a big difference to Carolyn. It changed how others responded to her and reinforced her good feelings and energy. Choosing to wear becoming colors gave her more personal power.

Clothes may not make the person entirely, but they sure do say volumes about you. And success builds on success.

Go for Volume

Expose yourself to high concentrations of eligible people. Increase your chances of finding your perfect partner by enlarging your pool of choices. Plenty of people exist to whom to be attracted. Unfortunately, being attracted isn't the same thing as matching on the 16 differences that make a difference. Attraction counts, but it isn't the whole story. Remember that you don't have to act on every attraction you have.

In the next section we're going to cover the advantages and disadvantages of the places to look for your perfect partner. There is, however, one place that really stands out when it comes to going for volume: the dating service. Here you have the opportunity to rapidly sift through hundreds, or even thousands, of serious people.

Look in the Right Places

This calls for action. Develop a strategy for exposing yourself to high concentrations of eligible people. Don't drift along waiting for your perfect partner to show up. They won't.

Generally, let selective others know you're looking and available and that you want their introductions to interesting people that they believe fit the description of your perfect partner. Why be selective about letting others know that you want them looking for you? Because you want others looking that will attend to your agenda not theirs. By that we mean, people that don't take care of themselves or follow our suggestions are going to hook you up with people more like themselves rather than potential partners that fit the description of those for whom you search.

By letting others know you're looking you enlarge your circle of choices and further establish intention within yourself.

More specifically, let's look at the places in which to find singles also looking for their perfect partner.

Places to Look

Different kinds of people go to different kinds of places. And people that have their head straight spend most of their time doing things they enjoy.

Look in places where people who have the same interests that you have go, and increase your chances of finding your perfect partner. Increase your pool of choices the most by going to places where high concentrations of eligible partners will be. Increasing your choices, also, dampens the impact of rejection because you know many others are there from which to choose.

Expend your resources – time, energy, and money – on places and activities that include potential partners. Proactivity and commitment to marrying the right partner require you to funnel your resources where it counts. Since we believe that having a great marriage sets the stage for success in the rest of your life, we believe that finding the perfect partner is at the top of the list of first things first.

Let's explore possible places you can go to find potential partners with your interests. Each place has its own possibilities and limitations.

Places where you spend a lot of time...
School

Benefits:

-Many single people your age; some with similar interests; College & Grad school good place depending on level of maturity

Limitations:

-Too young to know yourself and whom you should match
-Lack of experience managing emotions and relationship skills-High school - too young to know yourself, good for practicing dating

skills and getting to know and be friends
with the opposite sex

Because we're in school when we begin to have
an interest in dating and romance, school is the
obvious first choice for places to look. High
school and college offer you a practice arena,
but being young and inexperienced school is
best limited to getting to know others, learning
how to make friends and be a friend, and getting
to know what we do and don't like. School is a
time for experiencing many kinds of activities
and relationships, trying them on for size,
which helps you, get to know yourself.

Spend your time and energy during your
school years getting to know yourself. Pay
attention to what you like and don't like.
Participate in activities that you like and you'll
meet others that like the same activities. That
is, unless they don't spend time doing what
they like. Some people spend their time and
energy doing what others expect them to do.
You must learn to observe for those people and
observe the difference between them and those
that spend their time and energy doing what
comes natural for them. Find out what you like
to do not what others expect you to do and get
involved with others that can do the same.

Find out what the opposite sex is like.
Become friends with others. Polish your relationship skills. Practice dating.

In college, as you begin to concentrate
your efforts in major courses, get to know others majoring in the same or similar subject
areas. They will have similar interests.

As you get older and more experienced

you'll have a better chance to select partners that come closer and closer to your perfect partner.

Take your time. You have the rest of your life. College does offer the advantage of a concentration of single people, but you have to weigh that advantage with the possibility that you just don't know enough yet to pick the right person.

We're going to discuss decisions about sex more extensively in the next chapter, but we caution you to understand that you have a physical drive to have sexual relationships. Be careful to choose when you'll exercise that desire and be selective about having a sexual relationship. Having good sex is one of the most pleasurable activities you'll have as an adult. Save it for the most important relationship. Having sex deepens your attachment and bond to someone. If you have sex too soon, you'll end up attached to someone with whom you're incompatible, but you won't find out until it hurts to end the relationship or suffer onward. Nothing is better than happiness forever, but nothing is worse than misery for the rest of your life.

Don't have sex until your emotional maturity has reached a level of functioning in your best interest. When does that happen? When you have control over your responses to your feelings. When you can think clearly before you act. When you can be brutally honest about what the behavior of yourself and others is all about.

Kim came into therapy tearful and unhappy over the breakup of a high school romance. Jack had been her first love, her first sexual experience. Kim was in awe of this football hero that would surely be king of the prom. Unfortunately, she was so in awe that she didn't notice that he didn't return her respect and admiration. Most of the time he was engrossed with himself. But Kim's physical desire for sex got tangled up in her desire for affection and validation, so she found herself in over her head before she could figure things out.

Having sex with this boy in her high school class and then their breakup had Kim thinking of suicide. She was one of many that end up feeling suicidal as a result of relation-ships gone bad. Her emotional maturity hadn't caught up to her physical maturity. She could-n't handle so many conflictual messages her body and brain were giving her. She wasn't ready to make such important choices about sex and relationships. And don't kid yourself. Boys get tangled up in the same mess. Not as often as girls, but they get hurt over being dumped by their sexual partners, too.

Young men and women in high school and early college need more time. Many need more time than college provides. Our best advice is to save sex for a relationship that you think is with your perfect partner.

In this day, when college serves as a tran-sition from childhood to adulthood, we don't grow up as fast as past generations. We don't have to go out and make our way in the world until later. We have others taking care of us longer and we don't have to learn to make deci-sions based on who we are for much longer. But making decisions and thinking for ourselves is what gives us the kind of competence and high self-esteem that it takes to pick the right marriage partner.

Your age doesn't matter as much as when you know who you are and are able to behave in accordance. What does matter is being able to think for yourself. Whatever age you are when you learn to think for yourself and trust yourself is when you're ready.

Work
Benefits:
-People with similar interests-You and others have gained maturity-Meet new people

Limitations:
-Wide age range
-Many already married
-Dating coworkers has some serious drawbacks
-Breaking up is hard to do
-Can affect your career negatively

Once you're out of school and into the work world, your environment changes.

Looking for someone at work has disadvantages. People who work where you work may or may not have similar interests. The work place is also fickle about its support of coworkers who date and/or fall in love. Relationships are tricky enough without your boss and coworkers looking over your shoulder. While there may be coworkers with similar interests, you usually have limited numbers of people from which to choose, given that there's a wide variation in age, and the fact that many are already committed.

Breaking up and having to see each other every day is painful. Taking your time and dating without sex will lessen that possibility, but it still exists to some degree. Realize that working with someone with whom you're dating can change the dynamics of the work group. Others feel left out sometimes. If you date someone with higher or lower status in the work group the power structure of the group changes.

You must consider issues of sexual harassment when you contemplate dating someone in the workplace. The climate in which your behavior will be received is decidedly more risky than in times past. What if you reject someone and they pay you back with complaints of sexual harassment? What if you follow all of the rules of respect and friendly manners and your behavior is still received or interpreted as harassment? Dating in the workplace has become a serious risk. We're not complaining about real sexual harassment – don't do it. But circumstances can be distorted and misinterpreted and wreak havoc on your life.

Carolyn dated a doctor from the hospital in which she worked after her separation from her first husband. She tried to keep her relationship discreet, but hospital communities are like small towns. Everyone knows everyone else's business. The doctor she dated had more status at work and coworkers resented Carolyn's influence on him. The doctor enjoyed the influence he had over Carolyn and wanted her to carry out his orders over others' protests.

It was a mess and couldn't last. Many things were wrong with this relationship, but the dynamics at work were detrimental to the relationship and to Carolyn's work relationships.

A patient met her nine-year live-in partner at work. Their relationship has been on the brink of collapse on several occasions. They work in the same office and see each other all day long. Connie has two problems. Seeing each other at work all day gives them plenty to complain about at home. Connie gets accused of gossiping too much. Gene flirts all of the time. Look in the work place. Practice dating, but be cautious about serious dating with someone from work.

Get help from others to make the right match...

Friends
Benefits:
-Know you well
-Have similar interests
-Each know more people

Limitations:
-Have an investment in you and with whom you marry
-Have their own agenda
-Only know a few more people than you do

Family
Benefits:
-Know you well

-Each know more people

Limitations:

-Have their own agenda

-Have an investment in whom you marry

Introductions, with some advantages and many disadvantages, are an age-old way of meeting someone.

Introductions by friends or relatives can be successful, but only to the extent that they practice letting you be who you are. Most people have their own agenda and if they don't have their head straight can be more interested in matching you with someone for whom they approve rather than someone in your best interest. You enlarge your circle of choice by asking others to make introductions, but you must be selective about whom you ask. Ask only those that don't have an investment in controlling your life. The partner you choose to marry will have an affect on your relationships with friends and family so they want you with someone that doesn't threaten the status quo.

Remember that most, if not all of your friends and family believe that you have to work hard to make any marriage work. If that rule goes unchallenged, the people they choose for you to meet may not be a very good match for you. Unchallenged, that rule allows them to believe that anyone okay will be good enough. That's a set-up for failure.

Guilt from not conforming to your friends and family's wishes can add tremendous pressure to the dating process. Another benefit of getting your head straight and dating practice is that you increase your confidence about your choices and have no difficulty placing limits on others. As much as you don't want to believe that a friend or relative would want to see you unhappy, many would like to keep you on par with them. Or at the least, they don't even know great relationships exist.

Wes had quite an experience with an introduction one of his family members made to him. His brother-in-law worked with a young woman in Texas whom he thought Wes would like. Wes was fresh out of his painful eighteen-year marriage and hungry for some affection and companionship. He'd had a taste of excitement believing that it would now be possible for him to find a partner that would love him back, but he was vulnerable and longed for love; a set-up for disaster.

So Wes called Roxanne and attempted to get to know her over the phone. During the course of several conversations he decided that he wanted to get to know her better and wanted her to fly to Maryland. Working for an airline, flying was easy and almost free for Roxanne. But Roxanne wouldn't do it. She asked Wes to write her some letters. So he did. And Wes, being Wes, wrote of the possibilities of love and romance.

Two things happened that made this arrangement impossible. Wes's family was busy talking to each other coast to coast about how he keeps house and his looking for love. The husband of Wes's oldest sister was in town on business and spent the night with Wes. After staying with Wes, his brother-in-law told his wife who told their mom about Wes's messy housekeeping and she told his sister whose husband had made the introduction. From Maryland to Ohio to California to Texas. The bother-in-law that made the original introduction, a neat-nick, relayed the news to Roxanne. Roxanne and Wes had never met, but the family was already interfering with his relationship. When Wes tried to find out how Roxanne felt about him, she brought up the messy house.

Next, Wes's expressions of desire for love alarmed Roxanne and she showed his letters to friends instead of handling her thoughts and feelings directly with Wes. She publicized the proposed intimacies just like in junior high school. Here's a man who isn't afraid of intimacy and sharing – a man most women say they would die for – crashing and burning as punishment for his sins of unmanly openness. These events embarrassed and humiliated Wes and prevented any possibility of these two checking each other out. Of course, we're most grateful for the interference in the long run (rejection does you a favor), but this circumstance is an example of poor boundaries on the part of family members, Roxanne, and Wes. We'll talk to you more extensively about boundaries in the last chapter.

Romantic, intimate, marital type relationships are private. Marital privacy is what differentiates romantic relationships from other types of relationships. Mature marital partner discuss their intimacies and conflicts directly, between themselves. If they need to reach out for help, they contact professional help.

Complaining endlessly to others about their disappointments in love and marriage only continues the pain and solves nothing. Complaining adds another layer of hostility. Gossip can deepen emotional pain for everyone. Marital events and personal histories are not for discussion with others. It is up to prospective partners to learn all about each other and to form their own opinion about the other's suitability as a mate. And Wes's innocent trust in this potential partner and his family to keep his confidence and allow him to take care of himself in his own time doesn't work in the adult world. He was too quick to deepen intimacy before he'd established a trusting relationship. He was too open. He needed better boundaries.

More damaging is the possibility that such a match would only repeat the mistakes made in his first mismatched marriage. After all, family members were used to things the way they were, had only mediocre and poor marriages in their own lives, and had an investment in Wes continuing in the role he's always played in his family script. No matter how well intentioned people are, they still have their own agendas.

Please don't limit your search by confining yourself to this method entirely.

The Social Network
Benefits:
   -Increases you number of choices

Limitations:

-Hard to know who would match

Two books: <u>Love That Lasts, A Singles Guide to Finding a Great Mate</u> (Jongeward and Raffin, 1993), and <u>How to Find the Love of Your Life</u> (Dominitz, 1994), have adapted a technique from the business world that companies use to find the right employee for a job. It can help you find the right partner.

When businesses need to find the right person for a job, they often hire an executive search firm, sometimes referred to as head-hunters. The headhunter's first step is to make sure he understands what the employer wants, just as you need to specifically understand what you want. The headhunter begins search-ing by contacting people in his network who might know of people who fit the job or, more likely, know of people who might know some-one. What he's doing is dramatically expanding his contacts by asking each person that he con-tacts if they know someone who fits the job, or if they know someone who might know some-one who fits the job.

Make a list of all the people you know. After some thought, set up a referral interview with some of these people. At the interview, ask them if they know of any single people who fit what you're looking for. Get their help in locat-ing potential partners. Jongeward and Raffin have adapted this technique to what they refer to as a Social Network Party. They use this referral process to invite selected single people to a series of dinner parties hosted by their friends. This approach is good because only people who are selected get invited to the parties and, because of the ever-expanding number of people who know other people, the pool of eligible people that you can tap greatly expands.

We don't know anyone who has tried this method, but it sounds promising given the right circumstances. Wes contemplated using such a technique, but decided against it for reasons specific to him. He didn't have the furniture and equipment to host such a dinner or party and his housekeeping and social skills limited his desire to use this method. Being reserved and shy to some degree didn't lend itself to parties. However, after some dating and social practice he did become more comfortable in social situations.

Prerequisites for using this method would be an extensive network of friends, a high level of social comfort, an appropriate place, and furniture and equipment necessary for hosting parties. This method isn't for everyone, but if it fits your situation it can enlarge your pool of choices considerably.

Personal Ads
Benefits:
- Can specify what you want, the qualities you seek
- A large number of singles looking for marriage partners increases choice
- Relatively inexpensive
- Helps you restrict dating to only definite possibilities

Limitations:
- -Ads are too small to convey much information
- -Can run into some strange people - even dangerous people
- -Must screen carefully and as anonymously as possible
- -People may misrepresent themselves

The major disadvantage of personal ads is that it takes an enormous amount of information to decide whether to spend your time, energy, money, and emotional capital to go out with someone on a date. At least it does if you're using your dates to find your perfect partner and not wanting to spend your whole life on the process. The amount of information in a personal ad is miniscule. You need to have some idea of how well you might match, if you have some physical chemistry, and whether you'd be in any physical danger. That information is hard to get from an ad.

Only if you combine an ad with extensive phone conversations will you be able to know enough about someone to date them. You may spend a lot of time going out with people who aren't right for you, and you'll get discouraged and frustrated.

We've both known people that used personal ads to search for a partner. Getting responses wasn't a problem for them; only weeding through all of the responses was a problem.

Carolyn knew someone at work that used personal ads to find dates. She did find dates, but unfortunately, she'd started using ads because she couldn't get dates any other way. The real problem was that she was seriously overweight. We're not talking about twenty or thirty pounds overweight, but probably two hundred pounds overweight. This person felt protected by the anonymity of the ad, but once her dates learned of her obesity the possibility of further dates ended. You can only hide behind the anonymity of ads (and computers) for so long.

On the other hand, Wes met someone at the Crabtown Ski Club (an activity group in the Annapolis area) that decided to put an ad in the Washingtonian. Wes watched curiously while this banker, sailor, jogger was deluged with responses. And the responses came from a variety of professional women. Jim's problem was sifting through the responses to find appropriate dates. He actually set up a grid where he tracked the responses. We've lost track of Jim, but last we heard he enjoyed dating a multitude of women, although he hadn't settled into any one relationship. Wes thinks Jim was probably just interested in dating, not in marriage, because he believes that with so many attractive and interesting people from which to choose, doing so wouldn't be difficult. He may not have wanted marriage as much as he said he did. That would be a case of not matching your behavior with what you think and feel, which many people come to do after being hurt repeatedly in the dating marketplace. Or maybe he only said he was looking for marriage because he believed no one would date him unless he intended a serious relationship.

Personal ads don't contain very much information and the potential exists to use all of your time and energy up on people that won't match you. Given the time and energy it takes, we don't think personal ads are the way to go.

Computers
Benefits:
  -Great matching tool if someone would put together the right kind of database
  -Large pool of choices
  -Look in the privacy from the privacy of your home

Limitation:
  -Existing databases don't have the 16 differ- ences that make a difference as matching critera
  -Easy to misrepresent yourself
  -Geographical limitations
  -Most don't have pictures or videos, which will change in the future

Can the computer provide you with the kind of information you need to know whether to go out on a date with someone? Can the computer overcome the distance problem it presents because it can link you to most places in the world?

In the future we're sure computers will have video components enabling you to gather more information about someone as you talk to them. They'll also be able to connect you with people in your proximity. Until then, what computers have to offer is limited.

Nevertheless, computers do have tremendous potential.

The Internet and other services like America Online, Microsoft Network, CompuServe, Prodigy, etc. offer chat and news rooms in which to get to know others. Users frequenting chat and newsrooms usually have similar interests. The Internet also offers actual dating services which will match you with potential partners that list similar characteristics. Computers also offer a degree of distance and anonymity that can increase your sense of safety. That same distance, however, can also be your downfall. Sooner or later you have to have the courage to meet the person. Don't use the computer to hide behind. And that person could live a half a world away from you. You may begin an attachment that could necessitate a move or career change.

Carolyn has a group of women friends that believe computers only serve to reinforce social isolation. Since they don't use the computer they don't realize that computers actually enlarge your world considerably. They don't see how it's possible to actually increase your social and business contact through the use of a computer. And since people that use computers remain a mysterious group to them, they only believe what they've heard some others say – that users of computers are social isolates. We disagree with that. Of course, others can scam you in a major way. The ability to disguise your real self to others, to misrepresent yourself on the computer must be taken into consideration. Only being face to face with someone, over a period of time, can give you the kind of information you need to have about whether the person is who he or she says they are.

The potential for computer matching won't work until it offers regional matching to possible partners within driving distance of each other. That kind of a dating service would also need to follow our suggestions for matching to increase the rate of success. We think the potential is tremendous for matching purposes.

Singles' Clubs
Social GroupsBenefits:
   -Increase choice
   -Structured activities having fun
   -May have similar interests

Limitations:
   -Others may not be looking
   -Still hit or miss dating to some degree depending on what kind of group

At singles clubs you can meet a lot of people and have fun at the same time.

Lots of communities have a variety of singles' clubs. Some are not even restricted to singles. They've been so popular in structuring fun activities that many allow married couples and families to participate. Clubs usually have a membership fee for administration purposes, and a small fee for activities. The fees are often less than what you'd spend alone because of group participation.

Community clubs – such as our local ski club – provide planned activities for a variety of interests such as skiing, eating out, country dancing, sailing and motor boating, biking, hiking, and travel. Participating in a group like the ski club offers you the opportunity to try new activities with help, and exposes you to a group of people who enjoy activities you like. Social exposure reduces the risk of running into strange people. Strange people who may be harmful are exposed pretty fast. There may be a fair number of less than serious lookers due to the modest expense and ease of participation. You may run into those who say they're looking for the right partner, but may have little commitment to the process. They may not have done any of the head work necessary in order to know yourself. You may run into a fair number who are only partly serious about finding what we're talking about here: intimacy and a great marriage.

Wes joined the ski club and participated in biking and hiking, which he already did on his own. He also enjoyed sailing with the group; an activity he'd always wanted to try. And he met others that became friends and played bridge with him. He had a lot of fun participating in activities. He had mixed success in the dating department, but did get to know and date about 20 women over a year and a half.

Initially, he lacked the social skills necessary for meeting people in mixed groups such as the ski club had. One of the things he liked was the opportunity to practice social skills and become more confident about meeting and dating others. Plenty of role models were there to watch – both good and bad. He always had something to do, whether he had a date or not, which took some pressure off him to find someone right away. If someone turned him down for a date, he could go on to the next interesting person and if he dated someone once or twice and it didn't work out, he didn't have to feel bad for long because someone else came along to date.

Wes did feel his choices were still limited. He had some success, but still didn't meet exactly the right person.

After we started to date, Wes took Carolyn to a few of the ski club functions. Friends had told her about the ski club, suggesting she join, but she'd decided not to. Carolyn remembers thinking that many of the participants may not be serious about marriage, and she wanted a good marriage partner. She didn't want to spin her wheels dating people and find out later they were uninterested in marriage. Many people say they want to be married, but then act as if you'd have to trap them into it. Carolyn wanted to avoid head games.

So she went with Wes to a dance at Christmas right after they became engaged. And she didn't like it very much. Several women that hadn't seemed interested in Wes while he was looking were suddenly all over him. (Why is it that women that refuse dates with a man initially suddenly interest themselves in men they can't have? Sounds like a case for getting your head straight to us.) One actually came up to him and tried to talk him out of marriage. She stood next to the table where we were sitting and looked at Carolyn as if she was a small child displaying bad manners. She actually shook her finger at Carolyn. Men looking for a partner clamored to meet Carolyn. Even men Wes had known from activities. One doubted our engagement openly saying Carolyn didn't have a ring on. One thing is for sure. We attracted a lot of attention. Everyone wanted to know how we'd met each other.

Unhappy as she was at the dance, Carolyn agreed to go on a skiing trip Wes had already planned to attend. She'd always wanted to try skiing and this was the chance. Wes arranged Carolyn's sign up for membership and the costs of the trip.

We had lots of fun together on the trip, but the group was an awful experience again for Carolyn. (This time she did have an engagement ring on.) One man tried to get Wes to leave her alone with him and challenged Wes in front of her. Carolyn asked him if he thought she'd actually give him any notice at all after treating someone like he treated Wes. Another older – and mostly drunk – man became irate and actually got in Carolyn's face when she declined to make coffee for the huge group, saying she didn't even know how to make it for herself in a small pot. She asked to exchange the task for something else and was called all kinds of nasty names. We had a private room, but women crashed into it while we slept. Just like high school class trips. They even had a toga party. The last time Carolyn attended a toga party was in college.

So Wes liked the ski club because their activities gave him an opportunity to do things he'd never done before (he was a serious high school and college student and didn't get a chance to get partying out of his system). They gave him a chance to practice meeting and dating all kinds of people. Carolyn had already been through high school, and college fraternity and sorority parties. She just wasn't interested in the ski club.

Community Support Groups
Benefits:
-Can help work through issues from past relationships
-Many single people there

Limitations:
-People feel vulnerable
-Attractive, confident people are already out dating

Many communities have support groups for single with broken relationships, newly divorced, or widowed people giving them the opportunity to work through their issues in a group setting with professional/peer guidance and support. One national example of this kind of group is Parents Without Partners.

Community groups can give you support while you get your head straight. They also often provide educational speakers, and planned social activities. Their activities tend toward parties rather than physical activities. Most of these groups charge a membership fee and/or a fee for certain activities. Some lean more toward support groups, some more toward social activities. The main drawback to looking for a marriage partner here may be that it's too soon after an ended relationship. As a first stage, these groups can be wonderfully support-ive. Some may be better than others at offering exposure to potential mates. You may have dif-ficulty identifying people with similar interests.

Carolyn joined an actual therapy group after the death of her husband. She knew she would need emotional support in order to with-stand the loneliness and grief. She wanted to avoid reattaching herself to another man too soon. She'd made serious mistakes in choosing partners before and didn't want to do so again.

At first she used the group to help her grieve. She experienced many emotions while reviewing her marriage and her husband's death. She finished unfinished business from her first marriage – unfinished business that had prevented her from selecting a more suit-able husband on her second attempt. She learned so much about herself, many new cop-ing strategies, and experienced so much peace from getting her head straight that she didn't feel lonely most of the time. She learned to use her dreams to help her solve problems and to know herself better. She used the time to com-plete herself so she wouldn't need a partner for completion.

After almost a year, she began to yearn for another partner. She missed sharing life with a man. She missed a satisfying sexual relationship. Then she used her therapy group for the emotional support of beginning to date.

It never occurred to Carolyn to look for a new partner in her therapy group. But she did remember a flyer that came in the mail about a dating service. And the stability of the group and her life gave her the courage to begin looking again.

Wes joined a local church supported singles' support group called Single Again. Devastated from the end of his painful 18-year marriage he looked for the support of the group, as well as, an opportunity to find women to date. He learned quickly that most of the members of this group were too fresh out of relationships and too vulnerable for dating, let alone a relationship. Once he realized that the other members weren't interested in dating yet, he settled in to learn as much as he could.

This group met weekly to hear an educational speaker. Topics included handling divorce and death from many perspectives. After the speaker the large group divided into smaller groups for the supportive function of giving each member a chance to verbalize problems and feelings and get feedback from other group members and the leader.

Going to this group helped Wes realize that other men and women had much more difficult problems to overcome than he and encouraged him to get himself out into the dating marketplace. He also learned many important ideas for dealing with rejection and the unfinished psychological business of his marriage and divorce.

These groups are of great benefit to members that use their time and energy to resolve relationship issues from the past and move on toward more constructive behaviors in the future. They are more than likely not for finding a new partner.

Dating Services
Benefits:
- -Increases choice
- -Staff screen members
- -Only serious people will spend the money
- -People tend to have good jobs or they wouldn't spend the money
- -Helps you market yourself
- -Can date only people that are definite possibilities for a match
- -Anonymity unless both agree to meet
- -Always new people to meet
- -Have social functions for meeting people
- -Limits rejection

Limitations:
- -Number of members makes a difference
- -They don't all work the same
- -You should be able to choose dates yourself, rather than the dating service choosing for you.

Dating services can help you market yourself to large numbers of interested people in a thoughtful and meaningful way. Dating services exist at the local, regional, and national level.

Dating services have gotten some bad press, not at all like the experience we each encountered through the dating service we used. Yes, we're biased for dating services. At least good dating services and we want to tell you why.

Let us say, right up front, that the fact that you've decided to enlist the help of a dating service doesn't abdicate your responsibility for selective dating, for noticing undesirable characteristics or behaviors in those you date, and for ending any relationship the moment you recognize something is wrong. We've seen negative reports of some dating services that are no doubt true to some degree. Things like sales tactics used to make the sale. But we can't help but notice that the critics seem to rely on others to do their thinking. The complaints we've heard in the media about dating services repeatedly sound like their clients want the service to protect them from everything. You must take the responsibility for your life and your dating experiences. If you get your head straight, know what you want, have reasonable limits and boundaries, you will do quite well in most dating services. But some are better than others are.

We're especially partial to this method, because this is how we found each other. The dating service we joined worked for us. We were both attracted to the practicality of the dating service. Since we both worked, we just didn't have much time to spend looking. When we did have time off, we wanted dates lined up already, so that we spent our time getting to know people. We liked the fact that the process of identifying people to date provided us with lots of information. Since we had so much information, we didn't have to spend a lot of time searching for basic commonalties. There's value in the time spent in this process. In other words, we produced a lot for the time and effort given.

The dating service we used, Great Expectations, is probably one of the more expensive ways of meeting someone. So the question is, how much money should you spend on the most important decision of your life? The money was well worth it because it offered us many advantages. Both the screening process and the cost keep out some weird people. It doesn't weed out those that don't have their heads straight and only think they want a partner, but it does increase the person's commitment to finding value for the dollar.

The process of joining forces you to think about who you are and what you want. It gives you marketing assistance with a large group of people in the dating marketplace. The process is anonymous until both have read each other's profiles, and decided it sounds okay to meet. That cuts down on the sting of rejection. And you can learn quite a bit about each other before you meet. With so much information, it's easier to sort out those that probably aren't compatible and identify those that are. The process increases your ability to focus on people with compatible interests and life styles. The large pool of members concentrates your exposure to eligible men and women. By the first time you meet, you've already done what you usually spend many of the first few dates doing. This has advantages and disadvantages: it reduces the anxiety of first dates, but it also speeds up the process.

Speeding up the process can be frightening, because things feel like they're moving fast. In many cases they probably are. But they're moving fast because everything is working out so well. We had no trouble with this, but our family and friends just about went ballistic. They were playing by a different set of rules (not knowing or even considering that we did know much more about each other than they believed time would allow). We spent a lot of energy talking them through the fact that we knew we were okay. To give you an example, Carolyn's son started asking questions like: "Do you know Wes's favorite color; or his middle name?" Her son chose questions to demonstrate to Carolyn that she didn't know Wes well enough, given the amount of time they'd been dating. After all, if Carolyn didn't know minor things about Wes, how could she possibly know the major things about him? But Carolyn knew all of the answers, and gradually her son came to see that we did have enough information to make such a big decision as getting married.

We'll tell you how the process went for each of us.

Wes began the process about a year and a half before he met Carolyn. He went to the dating service after receiving one of their flyers in the mail. The practicality of the dating service appealed to him.

The night he went in to be interviewed and screened, and to interview the representative of the service, he got a sales pitch from an attractive female employee. Not realizing ahead of time how much the dating service would cost, Wes choked when he heard the price. Eventually the sales rep talked Wes into a lifetime (value for the money...) membership for little more than a one or three year membership. He paid the bill and left in some mental turmoil.

He thought about having just joined the ski club and maybe this was a costly mistake. He should give the ski club more time. By the next morning he'd talked himself into a panic about whether he'd made a bad decision. So he returned to GE. They told him he couldn't back out of the deal. Wes asked to talk to the manager. Again, he was told he couldn't get out of the deal; there was no cooling off period. Wes was finally consoled when he asked the manager if he'd get value out of the membership and was assured he would.

Next, he wrote a one-page profile of himself. Demographic information such as where he lived (the town only), his age, education, job, whether he had or wanted children, smoked, drank, religious preferences, and other similar kinds of background information filled the beginning third of the profile. The answers to three questions filled the rest of the page. Those three questions were: Who are you, what do you like to do, and what are you looking for? (You can see that, with some thought, you can cover our 16 differences to some degree in this one page profile). With a little help from the staff, Wes polished his profile into a sales masterpiece.

(See the examples Wes and Carolyn's profiles following.)

Wes's GE Profile

FACTS ABOUT MYSELF:
First Name: Wes
Code #:
Date of Birth: 1/22/48
Eye Color: Blue
Hair Color: Brown
Height: 6'3"
Weight: 210
Occupation: Westinghouse Electronic Systems
Where Raised: Florida, Hawaii, Illinois
Education: BS, MS Physics U. of Illinois, MBA U. of Maryland
Marital Status: Divorced
Smoke? No
Date a Smoker: No
Drink? No
Number of Children: 2
At Home? None
Date Someone with Kids? Yes
Do You Wish to Have Children? OK
Religious Affiliation at Birth: Methodist
Now? None
Religious Dating Preference (if any): Prefer not very religious
Racial Dating Preference (if any): White

WHAT I LIKE TO DO:

When I was in graduate school, I put 7,000 miles on a rail pass traveling through Europe. Zermatt Switzerland, London, the Bavarian Alps in Southern Germany, and the Spanish Riviera were my favorite places. I have driven and camped across the US several times. I vacation every year at my parents in Ventura, California: Universal Studios, Disneyland, Raging Rivers, and the Ventura Beaches are my favorite spots. I have also traveled locally. New York City makes a great weekend trip. I like first class movies. I like to ski, bike, hike, and play bridge. I belong to a health club and do aerobics classes and Nautilus for an hour and twenty minutes four or five times a week. I read the Wall Street Journal every day and several computer magazines. I like to watch TV and work on my computer.

WHO AM I:
I am affectionate and romantic. I like to hold hands. I like to snuggle on a couch, watching a good movie or listening to music. I am independent. I like my own cooking. I iron my own shirts and do my own laundry. I believe in hiring someone to clean the house. I am health conscious. I have never had a speeding ticket. I believe in individual freedom, responsibility, and small government. I have an excellent job. My kids are terrific.

WHAT I'M LOOKING FOR:
I am looking for what I think I can deliver in a long term relationship: good physical chemistry, common interests, good breakfast table

conversation, financial stability, character, integrity, loyalty, and good conflict resolution and communication skills. I want, and am prepared to deliver, a very high level of commitment. Trust, affection, friendship, and a sense of belonging are what I am looking for in a relationship with an equal partner.

Carolyn's GE Profile

FACTS ABOUT MYSELF:
First Name: Carolyn
Code #:
Date of Birth: 3/14/48
Eye Color: Hazel green
Hair Color: Dk. Brown/Auburn
Height: 5'2"
Weight: 124
Occupation: Supervise Emergency Psychiatric Evaluations in Emergency Room of a hospital. I am a Psychiatric Clinical Nurse Specialist
Where Raised: Muncie, Indiana
Education: MS in Nursing, 1979, Johns Hopkins University; MS in Nursing, 1988, University of MD at Baltimore
Marital Status: Widow
Smoke? No
Date a Smoker: No
Drink? Occasionally
Number of Children: 3
At Home? None
Date Someone with Kids? Yes
Do You Wish to Have Children? No
Religious Affiliation at Birth: Methodist

Now? I am deeply spiritual, but not fond of organized religion.

Religious Dating Preference (if any): Probably a Christian orientation or open minded.

Racial Dating Preference (if any): Caucasian

WHAT I LIKE TO DO:

I really like a variety of activities. I like quiet moments reading, listening to music, the fireplace, TV (some), videos, the beach, walks, light hiking, taking pictures, rainy days. I can be introspective at times. I am also a very active person that likes bench aerobics, working out, gardening, yard work, eating out, movies, trips/travelling, my work, some small parties, some large parties, go to the theater, ballet, symphony, museums. I like keeping my home comfortable and open to others. I like family gatherings. I would like to travel more. I like helping people. I really like watching football on TV (or in person); I am a Redskins fan! I like following the Orioles, but I'm not as much baseball oriented as I am football oriented. I like water/boating activities; I love the Annapolis/Chesapeake Bay area. I like nature and watching/feeding the birds. I like to keep a dream journal. I like relating to people. I like living comfortably and well. I like to follow investments and am interested in the market, but not extremely knowledgeable. I like taking good care of myself. I like holidays. I like to celebrate birthdays. I need a little alone time to keep centered. I like to be affectionate and romantic.

WHO AM I:

I am a woman, full of life. I like my life and myself. I like most other people. I am a deeply spiritual person, but not particularly religious. I am an optimistic person, usually happy and cheerful. I have enjoyed many roles: daughter, sister, wife, mother, coworker, friend, neighbor, student, teacher, and therapist.

WHAT I'M LOOKING FOR:
A man with which to share my life. I would like him to be spicy, tender, sweet, and successful. It would help if we had similar interests. I would like a mutually supportive, reciprocal relation-ship of equal partners.

(Can you see all of the similarities in our profiles?)
Now on with Wes's experience....

He had a few still photographs taken in casual and dress clothes, which went into a notebook in their library on the facing page of his profile. An employee interviewed him on video for about two minutes and that video went into the library.

Once a week or so, Wes went to the office and spent time in the library going through the female notebooks, which held profiles alphabet-ized by the first name only (no last names, no street addresses or phone numbers). He picked up to five names of women that fit the criteria he'd determined would guide him in his search. After getting those choices from Wes, a staff member sent each of his choices a postcard saying that someone wanted to meet them.

After the women had a chance to see his profile and video they could decide if they wanted to meet him also. Only after both agreed were they given each other's full name and phone number. It was up to them to arrange a date.

Wes remembers his reaction to his early dates. He immediately saw a difference in the women he was dating. They were a cut above others he'd dated. He was pleasantly surprised that so many professional women were members. He also liked having dates lined up on the weekends when he had time off instead of using his time on the prowl, meeting people by accident.

When he met Carolyn he knew his membership had been the best time and money he'd ever spent.

Carolyn started thinking about dating not quite a year after her husband's death. She'd begun to feel jealous about her friends being couples and wanted a partner of her own. After a couple of dreams convinced her she was ready to look, she remembered a flyer she'd tucked away about a dating service.

Upon her return from a trip to observe the one-year anniversary of her husband's death she located the flyer and made an appointment to go to GE. Her experience was different from Wes's, but just as positive.

Carolyn's experience started out positive because she didn't need a sales person to convince her to join. She'd already decided the money was worth it and she knew how much it would cost. She liked the practical process that gave her more control over those people she did

and didn't meet. Within an hour she left with a
signed contract and appointments for her pictures and video interview. She contemplated a
national membership – you can join with a one-
city membership, a few cities, or have a national membership, depending on where you want
to live and look. But decided against it because
she didn't want to endure long-distance dating,
and besides, she likes where she lives. Both she
and Wes had dual memberships in the
Baltimore and Washington, DC locations. We
could visit both libraries and increase the members from which to choose to eight thousand.

Carolyn approached looking through the
library differently from Wes. She took her time
reading through most of the profiles before she
started to select some men to meet. She'd only
picked one when men started picking her faster
than she could get around to picking herself. By
her third week into membership she had five
requests for dates.

Then she had to learn to juggle dating
several men, which she'd never done. The first
man she rather timidly selected turned her
down, saying she wasn't his type. After a
moment or two of feeling sorry for herself, she
dug into checking others out. There wasn't
much time for feeling bad. Someone else was
always waiting to get to know her. The therapy
group she attended helped her with all of the
issues that arose.

Her sixth week of membership, along with
a few other men, she got the postcard that was
initiated by Wes. When she saw his profile and
pictures she told her mom and aunt, who were

visiting, that he looked great on paper – almost too good to be true. She saw they had so much in common and he fit all of the criteria she'd set up for looking.

A few things interfered with an immediate connection. She was dating someone that she liked, but, until she recognized it, was playing head games reminiscent of high school. Her mother said Wes looked perfect, which triggered her life-long rebellion against her mom. He was a computer person (nerd). His father had been career military.

One-by-one she worked through the issues. She dumped the head game guy that thought the only way to catch a woman was to make them think you don't want them. He'd also exhibited some undesirable characteristics that led Carolyn to believe that he could be aggressive and abuse substances. She talked to herself and her group about the rebellion against her mom (unfinished business). The result of which is that she stopped herself from making any decision based on what her mother did or didn't want, after taking her thoughts into consideration. She had three long phone conversations with Wes that convinced her that this computer person was intelligent, social, and interesting. He had many interests in common with her. And he was very friendly and respectful. He wasn't guarded. He could share his thoughts and feelings openly and appropriately. She decided that since Wes wasn't military himself, and didn't seem to be unduly affected by having been ordered around most of his life (she did come to see it had affected him later, but not seriously). So she give him a try.

On their second date she decided Wes was her perfect partner. Fourteen weeks into her GE membership she'd found him and knew she wanted to marry him.

Dating services provide some measure of safety. Still, be cautious and use your head; think for yourself. Different dating services operate differently. How they set up dates has everything to do with whether they will offer you help, or become more trouble than they're worth. One thing we particularly liked was that we got to choose whom to date. You need to be free to use your own judgement about choosing dates. Dating services offer many benefits in your search such as, helping you clearly define what you want, helping you market yourself, preserving your privacy, and offering a concentrated pool from which to choose.

Given appropriate use, we're sold on them.

Professional Matchmaker
Matchmaking ServicesBenefits:
-Personalized help to market yourself
-Increases choice
-Screening for dating only good possibilities

Limitations:
-Expensive (beneficial in some respects, but limitswho can use)

We recently came across a book by Julie and John Wingo, At Long Last Love, (1994), which covers finding a partner and having a "meaning-ful" relationship. What interested us the most was the fact that they're professional match-makers. Their fees are quite high, but the services they offer are remarkable!

We don't know if other services like this one exist, but this is even more personally focused than a dating service with many of the same benefits. If you have the resources, they may be of help. We believe they try to match their clients among themselves.

Their matching criteria would have to be on par with ours to increase the potential for a great marriage rather than a marriage of convenience. They say an 80% match is okay. We say you have to match 80% or above on each of the 16 characteristics and can't have a bad match on any one of them. They have a much smaller pool of people from which to choose because not many people can afford their services. They do the matching. One matching characteristic for those that use a service like this is money. They have money; they are looking for money, looks, and style. They may be settling for less of a match overall to have those points match well. Is that what you want?

Good dating services offer you more value for the money and you have a much better chance of finding your perfect partner because of more members from which to choose and you do the choosing.

The Bar Scene
Benefits:

-Provides a social gathering of single people

Limitations:
-The people you meet may rely on alcohol to cope with social anxiety
-Potential partners may have a drinking problem
-Others may be looking for short-term relationships and sex rather than marriage
-Most use alcohol for recreation

We just realized that we left out the bar scene! That shows you what we think of it. Can you meet lots of people that are serious about finding a long-term marriage partner in a bar? Can you talk and exchange information in a loud, smoke-filled environment? Those are some of the big questions and we believe the answer is no.

Many people would like to believe that the cocktail hour is a sophisticated climate filled with sophisticated adults. Is that true? We don't think so. They're more likely to be people that can't share socially unless their anxiety is calmed.

Most of the unhappy patients that end up in therapy with Carolyn over relationships have bars and drinking involved somehow. They date people they meet in bars. When they get hurt, they return to a bar to look for the next partner. When they repeat this scenario over and over and still don't recognize why they keep dating unsuitable people, Carolyn wonders where their brains are in the whole process. Don't they understand that if they keep repeating what they've done to find partners they'll keep attracting and dating the same kind of people? People that go to bars to find dates all have one thing in common. They use alcohol for recreation.

Alcohol has so many drawbacks! When you tell people about the adverse affects of alcohol they believe you see alcohol as a moral issue, but it's really a physical poison to the body. It causes liver damage (because it's toxic) and vitamin and mineral deficiencies (because it's dehydrating and empty calories). Drinking alters thinking on the short-term and over time does lasting damage to the brain. Drinking damages developing fetuses during pregnancy and puts children in an environment that is hostile to their emotional development after birth. That's because blunting your feelings (alcohol blunts your feelings) prevents you from learning more constructive coping mechanisms for life and demonstrating them to your children. People that use alcohol on a regular, daily or almost daily basis lose sight of its slow and incremental damage to their function and their life. If you have to argue over alcohol and its very limited benefits with anyone, you're already under its spell.

Drinking isn't the problem initially; usually a sense of social inadequacy or desire to fit in is the initial problem. In which case, getting your head straight is the solution. Sometimes people use alcohol to medicate themselves for anxiety or mood disorders. In which case psychological and medical treatment is the solution. But over time alcohol itself becomes another problem. During the time you've used alcohol it has replaced your learning constructive coping skills, which leaves you at a loss if you quit.

It's hard to believe that you could ever find a partner with whom to be intimate in the sense we mean it in the environment of a bar. Maybe there are some exceptions, but not in general.

The first thing we'd suggest is an honest look at whether you need alcohol to feel comfortable enough to socialize. Are you fearful of rejection? Are you dealing with your loneliness by medicating yourself? Do you have a problem with alcohol? Do the people you're likely to meet at a bar have any of those problems? Finding a person for a safe and intimate relationship is complicated enough without adding alcohol to the picture. (By the way, some of the single clubs' social gatherings aren't much different from the bar scene).

Find appropriate methods of marketing yourself. Change your mind about the idea that you must pretend not to be looking. Change your mind that to be romantic it must happen by accident. Be the best you can be and look for your perfect partner with intention and purpose.

7

Dating with a Purpose

Decisions About Sex

Dating adds some intent to the romantic accident, but without purpose does little to help you find your perfect partner. Hit or miss dating wastes precious time and energy dating someone for weeks, only to find out well into a relationship that you don't have much in common. If you mistakenly have sex too soon under these circumstances, you deepen an attachment that will only bring frustration and pain in time. We want you to date with intention and purpose.

Stop and think about the reasons we date. Some people date to have a social life. Some people date to have short sexual relationships –

one night stands. Most people date to find the right person to marry. It makes sense that you match your style of dating to your goal.

If you're looking for a busy social life, you can date anyone that comes along. If you're looking for short-term sexual partners, you can date those that are likely prospects without much thought.

When your goal is a great marriage – and ours is – you must date with that goal in mind. To find the right marriage partner for you to have a great marriage you need to learn certain things about your prospective partner, right from the beginning.

To find your perfect partner you must date with the purpose of answering five crucial questions – the first of which is how well do you match on the 16 differences that make a difference? (Chapter 8 will guide you through all five of the questions.)

When we surveyed a group of singles we learned that 90 percent of them wanted to be married if they knew how they could find the right partner. But we also learned that the majority of those singles – approximately 65 percent – had one or less dates a month. And they didn't attend many social activities without dates either. Unless you have someone arranging a marriage for you, you must date to find the right marriage partner. In the western world we find our own marriage partners, so that means you have to get out there and date. Dating gives you the opportunity to get to know prospective partners and to know yourself better. Dating gives you the chance to master good social skills.

Dating Obstacles

If dating is so important, why do so many people have so few dates?

The major reasons people have few dates are fear of rejection and lack of opportunities to ask someone for a date. Many people also believe that meeting the right person will just happen, so they sit back and wait – the romantic accident. We hope we've convinced you otherwise. Your perfect partner will not fall out of the sky into your lap. We've covered increasing the volume of your dates in the last chapter. Here we want to discuss the fear of rejection and overcoming obstacles to dating.

Fear of Rejection

Rejection actually does you a tremendous favor. That's because someone that's rejecting you has noticed, that, for whatever reason, something about you doesn't match. Wouldn't you rather find that out sooner rather than later? Many of us are so intent on making the relationship work that we neglect to notice our differences. Unfounded loyalty just breeds misery.

No one likes to be rejected. Some of us have more difficulty with it than others. The difference between those that handle rejection constructively and those that don't relate to how you feel about yourself and how you think about rejection.

If you have difficulty with rejection, go back and review every chapter up to this point. Realizing how bad a bad marriage is and how painful divorce is can help you overcome your fear of rejection. It can help you appreciate rejection. Knowing yourself, acting like yourself with confidence, and liking yourself all help you manage rejection constructively. And when you market yourself and look in the right places, the increased confidence in yourself and knowledge that someone else is right around the corner will expand your ability to handle rejection. Do the legwork we've outlined for you and you'll improve your ability to withstand rejection and move on. Why in the world would you want to be with someone that doesn't want to be with you?

If you must, when you get rejected, mope around for awhile. Call your friends and complain. But don't waste too much time and energy on analyzing the situation. Spend some time on trying to identify what didn't match just so you'll have increased awareness about it, but don't waste your time putting them down to feel better about yourself. You're different somehow. That's all. That's enough. Some differences really make a difference. For the rest of your life. If you match on every difference that makes a difference except that the other person isn't ready for marriage, you have a difference that makes a difference.

But let's cover all of our bases. It could be that the other person doesn't know all of what we're telling you about finding your perfect partner. It could be that the person rejecting you is making a serious mistake. If you can account for a high degree of match on every difference that makes a difference, you must work on selling yourself to that person and convince them that they're making a mistake. If you like yourself, if you believe in having a great marriage, if you have confidence, selling yourself and your ideas about marriage will be reasonably easy. Selling a product that you believe in usually does most of the selling itself.

Master your fear of rejection. Think about rejection differently. See rejection as a favor to you and move on. Your perfect partner is looking for you, too. Don't deprive them of finding you.

Other Barriers To Getting A First Date

-not knowing enough about each other
-their fear that you're some kind of a creep
-they're already in a committed relationship
-stereotyped ideas about certain kinds of people
-the person acts disinterested when they aren't
-people are cautious because they've been hurt

The thing about barriers is to see them as a challenge, not as a signal to give up. It's possible to handle each one of these barriers so that you can keep going until you have enough information to make a decision about what to do. Indecisiveness often means a lack of information.

You can manage not knowing enough about each other by having a conversation or two with the person, or by asking someone that knows the person. You can best manage this by marketing yourself through a dating service, which helps you know more about each other from the beginning. It's easier to talk to someone who you know something about. Have a phone conversation or two and begin to get to know the person over the phone. Ask open-ended questions to draw the other person out. Close ended questions that only require a "yes" or "no" answer won't get you much information, and you'll end up frustrated. Open-ended questions, such as, "Tell me about the work you do," or "How did you decide to do the work you do?" will give the person an opening to share information about themselves which will lead to more things you can talk about. Developing a conversational style that includes open-ended questions is an important skill. It demonstrates an attitude of interest and curiosity about the other person, and enables the kind of answers that will begin to connect you with them.

Fear that you're some kind of a creep can only happen if the other person doesn't know you well enough. You can attempt to have a conversation with them in a safe (public) place or on the telephone, under non-threatening conditions. As they get to know you, their fear will subside. If you meet a stranger whom you want to know better, offer to have phone conversations with them, or meet them again in a public place for short periods of time, so you can get to know each other better.

Meeting and getting a date with a stranger is much harder than it is to be introduced to someone. When someone introduces you to a person, they can usually give you some information about the person. You have some basis for knowing the person isn't a creep. The best way to deal with this barrier is to meet people in a more structured manner, so you have more information about each other.

The person may already be in a committed relationship. Your best hedge around this problem is to choose from a group of people who have identified themselves as available. We don't believe in picking up strangers, because it leaves an awful lot to chance. You'll be well into a relationship and dating before you know enough about them to know if you even have a chance together as long-term partners. That's not to say that a great opportunity won't happen. If it does, and you want to initiate contact with someone you know nothing about, all you can do is look for obvious clues — like rings. If the person holds eye contact with you it's another indication that they may be interested, too. Asking a stranger has some risk to it from a few directions — most of all the possibility of wasting precious time. The worst that can happen is that they aren't interested, and since they don't know you at all, their lack of interest can't be due to you.

Stereotyped ideas about certain people usually have something to do with racial or cultural differences — or maybe age, or physique. Most of us have preconceived notions about others. Some are reasonable and some are not. Cultural differences have the potential to be differences that make a difference. Traditions and values grow out of cultural beliefs. On the other hand, someone's physique or slight age difference may not be a problem at all. You should treat anything that comes up in the way of stereotyped differences individually. Use the 16 Differences That Make a Difference to be sure about your match. Don't necessarily limit your choices by eliminating someone too soon.

Someone that acts disinterested may not be disinterested. It's common for someone shopping for something to act aloof at first, so they have some room to make a decision about what they want to do before they commit themselves. It's a protective defense. Be cautious and gentle here, but don't give up too fast, especially if you have any reason to believe they're just acting disinterested. But don't hammer away at someone who's doing everything they can to let you know they're not interested. This will take some judgment on your part; be sensitive to the person's verbal and non-verbal communication, and completely honest with yourself. Be sensitive to his or her social cues. On the other hand, there are times to take "no" for an answer instantly, like when the other person is turning you down for sex!

She said

Something like this happened to Wes and me

when we first hooked up with each other. As we told you, we met through a dating service. I got a card in the mail saying that Wes wanted to meet me. The only problem was, I had a couple of other men who had also asked to meet me, one of whom I was dating. When I read Wes's profile, saw his pictures, and watched his video interview, I liked him and thought we were a great match.

Unfortunately, I felt confused about what to do. I had started to date another man a few weeks earlier. I was having trouble in the relationship already, but some of my old behaviors had kicked back in and some old beliefs were confusing me. For one thing, I was falling back into the "making it work" routine. I "should" be able to do or say the right things and the relationship would work. Another old rule was about only dating one man at a time. I was having trouble knowing how to date more than one man at a time; I had never dated that way before. Also, my mom and my aunt were visiting me at that moment! My mom was telling me whom I should and shouldn't date, and I was reacting to her like I had so many times before. I was so angry with her for telling me what to do that I resisted listening to her. The problem was that she was right. If I made a decision opposite from what she wanted, my decision was still influenced by what she said, not what was best for me. I wrestled with this issue for a while, until I got my head straight about it.

I was lucky in several ways. I was in a therapy group just to maintain my center about these kinds of things. Talking the issues over in

the group helped me sort them out, and recognize what was happening. Also, even though I
was putting Wes off — the first time or two he
called I postponed making a date with him —
thank God he didn't let it stop him from trying
again. It took me a couple of weeks to get myself
thinking in my best interest, and he was right
there waiting for me. He hung in there because
I'd continued to let him know I liked him. In
fact, I think I was pretty up-front about what
was going on. I made it clear that my ambivalence had nothing to do with him, but that these
other things were happening. I'm sure, though,
that I upset him a couple of times. I'm so glad
he overcame any fear he had and kept going.

Remember: The hardest people to get a
date with may well be the best ones to get a date
with. Persistence pays.

Goals of the First Date

First dates are a lot like job interviews, except
that you're both interviewing and being interviewed. The object is to learn if you want to have
more dates and to get a second date if you want
one.

Even though you've done all of your
ground work, have made and are following a
plan to find the right person, have practiced the
skills for setting up and having a first date, you
can still run into people who haven't gotten
their heads straight. Precautions for handling
such people include having your own head

straight, having access to your feelings, and trusting your feelings. You can still run into those who present themselves one way for a date or two (or three or four), but later turn into people who are not who they seem to be at first, and who are into playing all kinds of relationship games!

Both of us ran into people that played games. One man Carolyn dated played hard-to-get, actually telling her at one point that you're not supposed to let the other person know you like them. It's an old rule and bored Carolyn quickly, reminding her of her high school days. How are you supposed to find your perfect partner if you pretend that you really aren't looking?

Wes ran into women that were seductive, but when it came down to having a relationship and sex, they didn't seem to really want either. When he found Carolyn and became unavailable, they were all over him. Something about already being wanted.

Games grow old fast and generally serve to frustrate the other person. Disguised and undisguised anger becomes part of the history of relationships with game playing. Game playing establishes power struggles in the relationship, where controlling the other person becomes the way of relating. Commitment issues get involved in this style of courtship and dating. Some people believe that they can win through intimidation and manipulation and some have learned to keep themselves at arms reach to protect them. For whatever reason others play relationship games, they prevent themselves from the validation of intimacy and they will keep you from the same. Avoid game players. If you're the game player, spend some time understanding yourself and why you've learned to prevent intimacy. Decide whether you want to continue walling off the pleasure and health that comes from intimacy. Practice letting down the wall and get your head straight. When you keep out the pain, you also keep out the love.

Patty grew up believing that men were scoundrels. Her mother had suffered at the hand of a few men and Patty inherited the legacy of all men are suspect.

Patty came into therapy when her 10-year live-in relationship ended. She was distressed and confused about what she wanted. Over time she recognized that she'd chosen to live with a man that feared intimacy. She'd chosen him because she also feared intimacy. For several years their arrangement suited her. However, over time she wanted more – she wanted the intimacy for which all of us yearn.

After working out the issues of ending the relationship, Patty found herself attracted to another man much more available to her in many ways. This new man was not afraid of intimacy and wanted marriage with an equal partner. He matched Patty in every way – except he was less fearful of intimacy. The new relationship went along very well until it was time to deepen its commitment and then Patty began to sabotage the fun and good feelings they had together. She came to therapy sincerely mystified about her behavior and wanted help to stop what she was doing. She didn't want to lose her new relationship – she wanted to marry this guy and maybe even have children. It was the first time she believed she'd found the right man to marry. The only problem was, would she let herself have what she wanted?

Fortunately, Patty had the determination and courage to work on the issues in her way. She could see what she was doing and she could understand where the fear was coming from. She began to realize that she'd have to bite the bullet and practice new behaviors, like disclosing her real thoughts and feelings, with this man, if she's to overcome her fear of intimacy. Slowly, she began to catch herself making indirect statements and not really saying what she thought and felt and slowly, she learned to stop herself. She learned to say, "wait, I don't mean that. I'm not sure what I want to say, but it wasn't that." Gradually, that statement became, " wait, I didn't mean that, what I meant was…." As she experienced the emotional safety this man provided – no ridicule, teasing, or intimidation – for what she expressed, Patty overcame her fear. She worked on increasing her self-acceptance to a more realistic level and she took a few more chances. What she learned was that this man didn't need to be feared at all. Patty gave up her emotional games and married her perfect partner.

Perfect partners don't play games and they don't frustrate your efforts to get to know them.

Dating Techniques

Two skills foster healthy relationships more than any others. They are relating to others from a win-win perspective and practicing the art of seeking first to understand and then to be understood. These two skills have been discussed in a variety of ways by a variety of authors, but we like the way Stephen Covey has discussed them in The 7 Habits of Highly Effective People. In his book, he's applied them to the business environment, but they apply to all relationships equally. Effective people have effective and satisfying relationships. Mastering these skills will help you relate to others in a healthy way. Mastering these skills will help you date with confidence.

Thinking Win-Win

You've gotten your own head straight and know that you're a vital, wonderful, deserving person. You've gotten in touch with your worth and dignity as a person. You may remember how crummy it felt to not feel this way about yourself. Congratulations if you've never felt bad about yourself, but you can imagine what it must feel like to feel that way. That's empathy. Being able to put yourself in another person's shoes and know how it feels is empathy. Empathy helps you relate to others in a healthy way.

The last thing you'd ever want to do is relate to someone else in a manner other than contributing to their feeling wonderful about themselves. You want other people to know the joy of feeling good about themselves. You, therefore, communicate with them in a manner which shows them you have the same respect for them as you do for yourself. This is thinking win-win! Wanting the other person's needs to be met as well as your own needs to be met is thinking win-win. Specifically, this means no put downs, maliciousness, or otherwise demeaning comments. Such verbal pollution undermines any trust you may build, sabotaging any chance for having the kind of great relationship of which we're speaking! Thinking win-win means you are as interested in meeting their needs and satisfying their wants as you are in meeting and satisfying your own. In win-win relating everyone's needs and wants are equal.

Of course the ultimate win-win is that you find your perfect partner and that the other person also finds their perfect partner. Win-win means letting go if you're not each other's perfect partner.

In marriage, if anyone loses, both lose.

Seek First To Understand Then To Be Understood

Something wonderful happens when you feel heard and understood. When someone affords you active listening, it makes even disagreeing palatable. Communication dramatically improves when you actively seek to understand what the other person is saying. Seeking to understand demonstrates respect. Seeking to understand allows the other person to exist in the relationship. And relationships involve two people not just one.

If you spend your time talking about yourself, or monopolizing the conversation, or getting your message across, the message you'll be giving, at the least, is that you're anxious and unable to focus on the other person, or at most, believe you're more important than the other person is. Being second fiddle in a relationship dominated by one person is boring, not fun, even destructive to you.

Seeking first to understand, then to be understood, means active listening. It means not only hearing what the person is saying, but identifying the feelings and meaning the words hold for them. It means displaying validation for what the other is saying just because they're saying it. Both partners need this skill. If you offer active listening, it will increase your success in creating the kind of environment in which trust will grow. Active listening creates a greater opportunity to learn who the other person really is.

This is how seeking first to understand then to be understood looks:

Dan: But that isn't the way it happened at all. I was upset with her so I tried to yank her towel off to tease her. To pay her back for what she'd just done.

Not seeking first to understand: You liar! You did not. You're mean and perverse.

Seeking first to understand: So you were trying to tease her and express your anger at her with some humor? You mean that you weren't trying to look at her body? Are you saying that you have no sexual interest in her, you were just peeved at her?

Do you see the difference? The person seeking first to understand still believed that the behavior was inappropriate, but realized that the intent of the behavior was quite different from the original interpretation or fantasy about the behavior. The person not seeking to understand is the only person existing in the conversation. No one else can have an opinion. And that belief and interaction has shut down communication. Who would you rather attempt to relate to?

The person seeking first to understand has established a trusting stance and can continue even to disagree with the behavior and suggest something more appropriate. They maintain respect with limits and boundaries, which is healthy. Since the person that did something offensive trusts them because they took the time to understand what really happened, they will most likely listen to the advice. Not so when they get shut down and forbidden to exist in the relationship.

The person not seeking first to understand spends much of their time misinterpreting the world and will be unhappy and dissatisfied with their life as long as they behave this way. Attempting to relate to someone without the skill of seeking first to understand and then to be understood is very unpleasant and unfulfilling for others trying to have any kind of a relationship with them. People that relate to others in this manner control communication to exclude anything that threatens their view of the world. It doesn't leave much room for you to be present in the interaction. Not seeking first to understand is not only poor communication, but it's an orientation that puts others into a box that only allows them to be whatever the person deems.

One last point. Don't forget that you get to be understood also. Don't leave that part out. After the other person indicates that they feel understood, it's your turn to be understood. Explain your own position and interpretation. Give them an opportunity to understand you. Clarify anything they may not understand to the best of your ability.

Interviewing And Being Interviewed

Most of us have been interviewed for a job. We don't know about you, but we've each had good and bad interviews.

Many people have some anxiety about whether others will like them or not. Many people have anxiety about meeting new people. Most of us forget that interviews give you information about the prospective employer, too. If you've worked through the previous chapters, we're hoping that your self-esteem, self-confidence, and sense of direction can help you overcome any shyness you may feel. You can do one more thing to help you be more comfortable.

When you go into a situation where you'll meet someone new, go there with the intention of finding out as much about the other person as possible. Doing so will help relieve you of the feeling that the meeting is all up to you and what you say. Putting your energy into knowing them can alleviate being worried about what to say and what others will think of you. Showing your interest in them will help them relax and tell you about themselves. Demonstrating interest tells them a lot about you and begins to create an emotionally safe environment in which trust can develop.

Even though you may feel some anxiety, make the call anyway. When you postpone doing something that you feel anxious about, you only increase your anxiety. When you go ahead and do whatever is making you anxious, you feel relieved and good about yourself. The worst thing that can happen is that the person will say no and somehow put you down. If they do that, they aren't worth dating. The next worst thing they can do is just say no they aren't interested. Hearing no may hurt briefly, but you'll live through it. Just move on. Or try again at a later time. The point is, make the call. Don't let anxiety or the fear of rejection immobilize you.

We know this is a bit old-fashioned, but for you women that are reluctant to initiate the first contact with a man in whom you have an interest, ask a friend or relative to make the introduction if at all possible. We don't believe that all men must be challenged with a chase, but some men do like the challenge, and some women just feel more comfortable not making the first move. If you know a man that seems to have a good match to you on the 16 differences, don't pass up meeting them just because you're reluctant to make the first move. You may miss any opportunity of meeting them and what a waste that would be. In that case, take the initiative.

Beginning to date someone is like interviewing and being interviewed. You need to learn certain information about each other in order to decide whether to have a relationship or not. Conducting a good interview is a skill. Being good at being interviewed also takes skill.

Interview the other person by working your questions into the general conversation. It's more interesting than a structured list of questions. Keep the 16 differences that make a difference in mind to guide your conversation. Don't try to learn everything at once. Some of the questions are more appropriate to discuss early.

For instance, what kind of work do you do or do you want to do? What made you decide to do that kind of work? – lead to information about work, educational ambition, lifestyle, and energy levels. What made you decide to work for the company you work for or go to the school you go to? – leads to those answers, but also information about where they want to live and how they want to live. What do you like to do in your leisure time or for fun? – answers questions about leisure interests, energy levels, climates they like, and gives you information about what you can do on dates for fun. The list of 16 differences that make a difference can guide you during your initial contacts and dates giving you purpose and direction.

Save your questions about children and sex until you've established some trust and rapport. Volunteering the complicated answers about why previous marriages or relationships ended can also be too much before you establish trust. Forcing intimacy doesn't work. Intimacy must develop at its own pace, over time. Dumping too much private information on someone is a real turn-off. Spend your first date learning enough to know whether you want a second date. Build a history; build trust one day at a time.

Don't make the other person pull information out of you. Offer information appropriately. Help them turn closed-ended, yes-no questions into open-ended questions. Find a happy medium between stingy information and too much information, too soon.

Trust

Intimacy requires trust. To be trusted you must be worthy of trust. Things you can do to increase your ability to be trusted:

-Show you trust yourself
-Accept others as they think and feel with
 appropriate limits and boundaries
-Respect wherever they are in their lives, you
 don't have to stay with them if they don't
 match you
-Think win-win
-Seek first to understand, then to be
 understood

You can demonstrate trust in yourself by back-ing up what you say with action. When you lis-ten to yourself you demonstrate that you believe yourself. By accepting them we're not saying you have to spend your life with them. We're saying that it's okay for them to be wher-ever they are. You don't have to stay with them.

Trust requires a match between what you say and do, in other words, honesty about who you are and what you think and feel.

When questions arise about subjects you don't want to discuss until you develop more trust, have some honest simple answers pre-pared. Offer the first level of understanding, and leave the door open for future discussion. Save the intimate details for later. A frequent exam-ple would be, "Why did you and your Ex break up?" The appropriate answer for the first date is that you outgrew each other. It's always the truth! But it leaves all of the details about spe-cific conflicts out until you've established a trusting relationship with the other person.

Wes ran into trouble a few times because he was so open and honest right away (an exam-ple of loose boundaries). We're not saying to be dishonest, but to save intimate and private details until later. Another example has to do with learning about each other's sex drives. It's not a subject to jump right into! There are clues, though, that can give you some of the information you need — at least enough to know if you want to keep going. Some of the clues are the age the person is in relation to whether they ever married, how involved they are in their children's lives, and whether they seem warm and interested in you versus cool and guarded. How much time does the person have for sex, given the interests they name? You can sense whether their life is jammed to the rafters with diversions, or if they have some open spaces where sex could fit in. This is an area where complete access to your thoughts and feelings, and believing what you think and feel, can come in handy. There might also be a place and time for some lightweight early discussions about having children and methods of birth control, which could offer some insight about general attitudes about sex.

Take Your Time

Be patient! It takes time to establish trust and intimacy.

Be enthusiastic! Your date is going to feel good if you're enthusiastic and show interest in them. Don't pretend, though. It's important to be genuine and it's easy to pick up if you're not. Enthusiasm doesn't have to be frantic. An active interest will do.

First Dates

Don't forget about phone calls. Phone calls are good ice breakers. You can begin to find out about some degree of matching before you even go on the first date by talking on the phone. If you have some phone conversations before your first date, much of the anxiety of the first date will disappear.

He said

My first date with Carolyn was probably the best first date that I ever had. This was partly because of the fact that we belong together, but also because of the three phone conversations that we had with each other.

After talking to each other on the phone and getting to know something about each other, it will be reasonably easy to decide what to do together. If this is difficult, you may not have much in common and we caution you that this is a red flag. Pay attention and don't just make do. If you don't have plenty of similar interests, watch out!

Sometimes one will have an interest that the other has never experienced, but sounds like fun, or is something they've always wanted to try. That's less of a problem than not having an interest in something. It'll give you an opportunity to open up your experiences and develop new activities.

Pick something to do that will offer you the best opportunity to relax, have fun, and talk more. Planning in this regard will offer you both the best chances to have a successful first date. And first dates are a big deal! No matter what you do, there will probably still be a certain amount of anxiety the first time out. Feeling fear doesn't mean to quit — it means to have courage. Just get on with it. If you've done all the groundwork we're talking about, you'll have more inner confidence and self-esteem, and this process won't be so difficult. It'll also be easier to walk away from if something isn't working out right.

He said

Who pays on the first date? I had some trouble with this when I first started to date. If the man pays for the date, does the woman think he expects her to repay with sex?

I worked out the issue of who pays in a simple way. I always assumed that I was going to pay for everything on the first date. If my date raised the issue of splitting the bill, that was fine with me. But I wanted to communicate in a simple way that money was not an issue. Finding the right partner is such an important task that spending money on dates was fine. I found that the women I dated were generally happy with this approach. Interestingly, in several cases where our relationship had progressed beyond first dates and the women started picking up part of the tab, they soon broke off the relationship.

She said

When I started dating I was much more con-scious about what I was doing than I'd ever been before. I'd worked my way through the process we've been describing. Being in a better place mentally, emotionally, and physically than I'd ever been before — even knowing all that I'd learned over time — I still had some of the prob-lems we've described to you.

I felt excited and nervous. I reminded myself to use all of the resources that I had to keep myself centered and focused.

I enjoyed the process of looking through the library at Great Expectations (GE) – the dat-ing service I joined – to identify prospective dates and potential long-term partners. I had good relationship and dating skills, so I was in good shape for the adventure. I have to say, in the grand scheme of things, it was a wonderful process, and relatively painless. It didn't take long either. As I look back, I believe that the more you follow the process we've described for you, the easier and smoother it'll be to find the right person to marry.

When I agreed to meet Wes, GE let him know that I wanted to meet him too. They gave him my phone number. He called me quickly, and he showed interest in getting to know me from the beginning. He never left me guessing – not so with some of the other guys I met. He persisted, even when I resisted initially. We set a date together, mutually agreeing on what to do and when to do it, and then he called me several times during the week before our date. During our phone calls we balanced asking for and giving information to each other. We talked easily together; some of the calls were quite long.

By the time Wes picked me up for dinner and a movie, we knew a lot about each other already. And when he arrived, he was funny and playful. It was Halloween time, so he showed up with a patch on his eye and other pirate gear. It made us laugh and broke the ice. It also showed interest, creativity, and his wanting to make an impression. I loved it.

We went to a restaurant I'd wanted to try. It turned out to be a great choice — the food was wonderful. We had a chance to talk face-to-face for the first time, which also went well. We both were comfortable with each other.

After dinner we walked a short distance to the movie theaters. (Normally we'd exclude a movie as a first date because you can't talk enough. We'd talked so much already it was like we'd had several dates. And we both love to go to the movies. In our case going to the movie was okay.) The movie was the Joy Luck Club. I was impressed that Wes had picked a movie about mothers and daughters. And the movie gave us plenty to talk about afterwards. Going up the tall escalator, Wes managed to get his arm around my waist in an affectionate way. It startled me, and I said, gently, "slow down," but I did enjoy his affection. I've never forgotten it, and he still does it when we go to that movie theater.

We drove back to my house. He wanted to

come in and he wanted to spend more time together over the weekend. I put him off, because I was still wrestling with some of my issues. But I did have a wonderful time with him. I felt comfortable with him, and I wanted to go out with him again. My aloof attitude was an attempt to buy some time. I told him I'd call him over the weekend because I had plans. I waited until the weekend was almost over before I called him — again, my indecision. (Every time I think of waiting to call him I feel bad. I know it hurt him. I'm just glad it didn't stop him.)

So I did call him, and he wasn't home. I left a message and he called me back the next day. We made a date for the next Friday after work for dinner and a movie. By then I was becoming clear about the other relationship, and about the fact that I liked Wes better than anyone else; I liked him a lot. I kept the next weekend free so we could spend more time together.

We went on our second date. When we got back to my house, I invited him in for a while. I told him I'd kept the weekend free, but guess what? He'd already made plans for Saturday and Sunday! I felt bad, because I'd put him off before, and I didn't blame him for making plans. But I was disappointed and worried that now he'd play games with me. He didn't though. When he got back from his bike trip on Sunday he called me. I invited him over, and we made a fire in the fireplace, listened to music, and talked some more. It was a wonderful evening.

He called me the next day, and I made it clear to him that I liked him a lot, and I wanted to keep going. The next day I got flowers at work from Wes. I loved them and I felt good about him. We made plans to see each other Wednesday, and we haven't been apart since.

He said

I find myself alone, wrecked upon the sands of divorce. After the break up of a 20-year relationship in a family with two children, I found myself, at 44, looking for a new long-term partner.

I consider myself to be a romantic guy in the sense that I always believed in the possibility of a great relationship. From my first marriage, I knew what I didn't want, having learned the hard way. Unfortunately, I had some doubts about whether I would ever find the right person. When I looked back over my past experiences with women, my efforts had been, on the average, highly unsuccessful, with a number of dismal periods. I had doubts about myself. Was I really attractive to women? How would I do in bed, given my past failures? But I didn't want to live alone and without a sexual partner. It was too awful to contemplate. I knew that I was a nice guy, not what my ex-wife believed. I had a good job, with stable financial prospects. So, I made finding a long-term partner my first priority with both my time and resources.

I wish I could say that I thought things out and came up with a logical and rational way to approach finding the right partner. I didn't. This book would have helped! My first idea was to try to find someone at work. I figured that someone who worked where I worked would have a good job, and be talented. Next, one of my relatives tried to set me up with a woman in Texas. Then I joined Single Again (a local support group for new singles) followed by the Annapolis Crabtown Ski Club (a social group for singles and couples) and Great Expectations (a dating service). As each step failed to produce the desired result, I went on to the next. I skipped the bar scene because I don't smoke and drink and I felt that it would be unlikely that I'd meet the right long-term partner there. I didn't try the personal ads, but I seriously considered it; and I have a short story to tell about that later.

I got a date with Kay (names changed to protect identity), a secretary at the office, whom I've known for many years. Kay was tall and thin, with rich, long black hair and white skin. She used to model some on the side. We had worked closely. There was always some underlying physical chemistry between us, but because we were both married, nothing ever came of it. She had a son. When her husband switched from working nights to working days, they discovered that they didn't want to stay together. I found out later that it was partly due to her being involved with other men; so they got a divorce. She then married a manager at work, but that didn't work out either. He was controlling. And they both had kids living with them that created conflict and broke up the marriage.

I heard all about Kay's former marriages on our first date. We decided to go to dinner at a restaurant in Annapolis. Things didn't start out too well when I couldn't find her house. I wandered way off in the wrong direction. She had to come and get me when I called from a pay phone. Since I had lived in the area for fifteen years, the fact that I couldn't find her place after she explained it to me was fairly significant.

We went to the restaurant. For some reason, I had this idea that I should be completely honest with her, that I should tell her enough about myself so that she would get to know me. I told her a lot about myself. I guess I wanted to be up front with her. But it made the first date too heavy. Later I decided that the best first date strategy is to make things as light as possible and to try and focus on having fun. Sometimes this is difficult to do if you have to face probing questions about your past marriage such as: "Why did you break up?" If I said, "Well, she hated having sex with me, and she thought I wanted it too much." How would the rest of the date go after such honesty?

On this first date, I got into trouble with sex several times. We'd been having a fairly serious discussion about relationships. Kay asked me what I liked, and I said that I liked sex. This remark somehow got turned into the idea that I was taking her to an expensive restaurant and paying for her meal, and in turn, I expected her to go to bed with me. Of course I wanted to go to bed with her. I always wanted to go to bed with her. But I didn't expect to "buy" it. I tried to talk my way out of this. I wasn't entirely successful, because at the end of the date, when I brought her home, she asked if I wanted her to pay for half of the dinner. I said no.

After dinner, we went back to my place because her son was home and we'd have more privacy. This was a big mistake. My place was still full of unpacked boxes from moving, and there was no furniture. She liked to smoke and drink. I didn't like to smoke and drink, but I stopped on the way home and got a pint of vodka. When we got to my place, since there was no furniture, and the TV was in the bedroom, we went and sat on the bed and tried to watch TV. She sat on the end of the bed and smoked and drank. I sat watching her, and trying to figure out if I was going to get to make-out any. No such luck. She finally had enough. I took her home. She never went out with me again.

I learned some more about first dates the hard way. And we weren't right for each other. I faced a dilemma that came up again and again: what to do when you find someone that you're physically attracted to and want to sleep with, but you know that you're not good long-term partners? A short-term affair may be the answer, but you run the risk of catching something and getting distracted from your primary goal. Besides, the emotional fallout is horrible when you stop seeing a short-term bed partner to move on.

In chapter six we told you about my trials by fire when my brother-in-law tried to fix me up with a coworker. What a disaster that was. Feeling hurt and humiliated didn't do much for my self-esteem. I learned to handle things myself from then on.

My "affair" with Roxanne (chapter 6) shows the kind of emotional roller coaster that can be part of the romance of finding the right partner. I was literally intoxicated by the prospect of being in love with someone who was in love with me after all those years of rejection from my ex-wife. I felt embarrassed, shamed, rejected and depressed when the smoke and dust settled. I still feel a little hurt even now when I think about it. The most serious problem from these feelings is that they can cause you to lose confidence in yourself. This can slow down your search for the right partner, and make it more difficult to be yourself when you really need to be. My solution was to pick myself up off the floor and hurl myself back out in the dating world as soon as possible. Something else I realized, only later, was that most people have been dating before, and many of them have had some rotten experiences with the opposite sex. Assuming you've found the right one, it may take you a while to get past the protective walls they've built.

I joined Single Again. Single Again is an organization whose goal is to help people who have come out of marriages and relationships with the emotional problems associated with splitting up. When I joined, I was unhappy with my situation, lonely and miserable, but mostly I joined because I thought I might find the right partner there. After all, everyone who went there was single.

After I'd been going for three or four months, the director told everyone (but I think she specifically focused on me), that Single

Again was not the place to find the right long-term partner. I think she was right, although a number of people did find the right relationship there, and I actually dated three or four women from there, one whom I liked quite a bit.

Single Again was good for me because it helped me work through some of my issues with my divorce. I felt better. Mostly I found out that I was in good shape compared to most people and that helped boost my confidence.

Single Again met once a week at one of the local churches. There would be an opening session or speech about a divorce related topic and then people would split up into small group sessions.

One of the most helpful lecture type sessions for me was one called "The Six Divorces". The first kind of divorce people have is the dissolution of the legal agreement which they have with the State that makes them married: a piece of paper. But getting unmarried is much more than just changing one's legal status on a piece of paper. The second kind of divorce is one of splitting up joint property, deciding who gets what. People often fight for years over things like a set of old records each one wants, something the director of Single Again said she did in her divorce. The third kind of divorce is for people with children. Over the rest of their lives that ex-spouse will always show up at weddings, funerals, graduations, and the like. The fourth kind of divorce comes about when you've finally untangled yourself emotionally from your ex. Emotions after a divorce tend to look like cooked spaghetti, tangled in a ball. It takes a long time to adjust emotionally to the end of a 20-year relationship. I can't remember what the other two kinds of divorces were. The point was that divorce is complicated and multilevel.

There's more of a lesson here than how to manage the emotional heartache and stress of splitting up with a long-term partner. What's especially important is to recognize how sad and stressful and unhappy a bad ending to a long-term relationship can be. It's especially painful when you contrast a bad relationship with the joy and happiness flowing from the right relationship. And once you realize this, you take a lot more care to find the right long-term partner.

I joined the local Ski Club. I wasn't making any progress finding the right partner at Single Again, except that I had worked through some of my problems. I decided to join the Ski Club. I wish I'd thought of it sooner, but it took me a while to find out that such a group existed. The Ski Club was set-up by people who wanted to ski and get group rates, but eventually it became a singles' club with scattered couples. At this point I had decided that I needed to find someone who liked to do the things that I liked. The idea was to go to a lot of fun activities and meet people with common interests.

In addition to skiing, the Ski Club goes sailing, biking, hiking, dancing, partying, and drinking. Each month's group meeting gives people a chance to sign up for activities published in a newsletter. I did some wonderful things with them, and at one point I signed up for almost every activity they had.

Sailing on the Chesapeake Bay was spectacular. Ski Club members pay a nominal fee for an activity, which has no real expenses such as hotel rooms or airline fares. The fee to go sailing is $5. My first adventure was an evening sail on a small boat owned by Jim. There were five of us: Jim, three women, and myself. Bea, a tall thin blond about my age; Rachel, a chunky real estate agent who brought terrific food on trips; and Mary, a pleasant woman, but to whom I wasn't attracted.

Jim was an interesting character; he was a divorced banker with a sailboat and a house with water access to the Chesapeake Bay that had a dock to moor his boat. He was either looking for a new partner or just looking to date a range of women. I could never figure out which, because I knew he was dating some first class women, but hadn't settled down. He was bald, thin, a runner, and a gentleman. I was envious in the extreme; but he'd had his problems with women too.

He told me a story about how he'd put an ad in the Washingtonian singles section to try and find the right woman. He wanted someone to run with him, among other things. His ad said he lived in Annapolis, that he was a runner, and that he liked to sail a lot. This ad, as you might imagine, produced a huge number of responses. The hundreds of letters overwhelmed him. He laid out all the responses on a big sheet of paper in a grid-like pattern. Most of the people didn't interest him. Surprisingly, there were a number of high caliber professional women, including several doctors, who responded, and he got some good dates. He also had a couple of dates with women who didn't match up in person with what they'd told him. He would show up at a restaurant, be totally surprised at what he saw, and run for cover.

On this particular evening sail, we all met at Jim's house. We made a short drive down to his dock, got on the boat, and, because there wasn't much wind, motored on out to the bay. It was stunningly beautiful. The Magothy River was a mile or two wide with green tree covered shores and led to the Chesapeake Bay. After three or four miles, Jim shut down the motor, and we set the sails to catch the light breeze. Sailing down wind, the boat moves with part of the speed of the wind, and there's almost no noise. Looking at beautiful scenery and talking is a great way to get to know people.

I liked Bea. A friend of mine had told me that he went out sailing with a group called Singles on Sail, and that everyone wound up swimming with no clothes on. Frankly, I found that pretty exciting. I wasn't expecting that with this group, and it surprised me to find the conversation turning a little risqué. Bea was the one who was feeling a little lustful. Although I later learned that Rachel, the real estate sales person, could talk sexy too, after she initiated a picnic table, mixed company discussion about men's penis sizes. Bea told us the story of her last hot tub party that resulted in several nude bodies in the tub together. It sounded pretty exciting to me.

After sailing, I asked her for her phone number, but she wouldn't give it to me, saying that she wasn't that kind of girl. I guess she felt that I wanted to go to bed with her based on the way she'd been talking, which was true. I looked up her phone number in the Ski Club phone directory, though, and called her anyway. She had two kids, and had been divorced for at least ten years. I always felt a little leery of someone who looks so good but has been single for so long. There has to be a reason. In any case she wouldn't go out with me. Most likely she was acting the way that she did to flirt with Jim, whom she considered the real catch.

DATING TIP: sailboats are a great way to meet women, especially if you're the owner and captain.

My next sailing trip was a three-day weekend up the Chester River on a 27-foot sailboat that sleeps four. We sailed across the Chesapeake Bay from Annapolis and up the Chester River. At night we rafted up with the other boats. Again, we sailed the next day, rafting up that night. We sailed home the next day.

Four of us were on the boat. Myself; Paul, the captain and owner with a house on the water, divorced, over 50; Bob, a single man about 50 who worked for the government but refused to talk about what he did; and Phyllis, about 40, who was an excellent sailor with a pretty face and nice legs. But, and this was always the big but with women like her who were attractive and pleasant to be around, she'd never been married before. There had to be a reason.

We all brought food, except the Captain, since he was supplying the boat. On this

Saturday in May, we loaded up the food, clothes, and sleeping bags, cast off, and motored down the Magothy River past the houses on the shore surrounded by trees with their docks and sail boats. The wind was up on the bay with white caps, blowing 15 or more knots. It was a great day for sailing, with blue sky and just the right amount of wind.

At the mouth of the Magothy, just north of the Bay Bridge, the Captain checked the Loran navigational system for our current location, and a nautical map of the bay for our destination. He punched the coordinates of a point at the mouth of the Chester River into the Loran, and it gave us a heading.

Out on the bay, the waves picked up size, and I started to get seasick. We crossed the bay, tacking back and forth, and at the end, motored up the Chester River to the rafting point. By the time we were all there, there were eight boats, including a powerboat.

Eight boats tied together side by side, far away, it seemed, from civilization. It was a party, with barbecue grills swung out over the sides of the boats. I went from boat to boat, snacking on chocolate covered strawberries and talking with people, looking for the right woman. I've always been rather weak on party skills, saying hello and striking up a conversation. Most of the people at the ski club are friendly, so I was able to do what other people who have good social skills do, and that's practice being with people, finding out what interests they have and talking about them. Unfortunately, I still found that many of the women were not really looking for a long-term partner. They wanted to have fun, but they didn't have the same goals I had. Later, I was able to identify the people who were serious quickly.

Phyllis was not one of the serious ones. She had a hammock she set up on deck in which she asked a number of men, including myself, to join her, sitting face to face straddling the hammock. She had nice legs and it was quite stimulating, but I couldn't figure out what she was doing. Her signals weren't clear. So, I didn't do anything.

Sleeping on the boat was like camping out. It was wonderful, except that I slept alone in a sleeping bag inside the torpedo tube that ran under the starboard cockpit seat. Paul placed a bed on top of the dinner table booth in the center of the sailboat. Phyllis slept in the forward cabin, alone. Bob slept out in the open on the aft deck. In the morning we cooked scrambled eggs. It was great.

The next day we sailed part way down the Chester River. But there was no wind, so we decided to just head for the next raft up where all regrouped. This time I went swimming along the shore, past a boat anchored in the distance, and back. I went from boat to boat talking to the skippers about their boats. The technology and the money spent on these boats fascinated me. The automatic pilots, wind indicators, speed indicators, radio, and navigational aids were fascinating. The speed indicators used the Loran radio signals or the satellite GPS to electronically calculate the true speed over the land. While sailing, you could tell what direction you were going and how fast. The largest boat there, a 42 footer, was bought by the captain from the Naval Academy, and he was actually living on it. It had a shower, which the women loved.

The next day we sailed down the Chester River and back across the bay. The wind was up big time. Going into the wind the water crashed against the bow and the spray flew back. I got seasick.

I went on another two day sailing trip later in the season, across the bay to a marina. This time, one of our crewmembers was a woman in her early 60's, Ellen, who had spent a lifetime sailing with her husband who was now, unfortunately, deceased. We had some great conversations about finding the right partner.

It took me slightly over a year to find Carolyn. During that time, I went skiing with GE members. I went to several GE sponsored parties. They were wonderful. There was good music and places for people to talk. There were always many dressed up and attractive people at the parties, a concentrated pool of people who wanted to find the right long-term partner. I went to two parties, and got dates with two attractive women. I normally have a tough time with parties, so this was good for me.

Rejection. I asked out dozens of women over the course of the year I was looking for Carolyn, and a fair number of them rejected me.

I have mixed feelings about being rejected. It hurts, especially when someone who you feel would make an excellent long-term partner rejects you. What's the best way to deal with

rejection? To me the answer is simple but not
easy. First, focus on being the best you can be.
Exercise and work out, lose weight, eat right,
get your head straight, dress sharp, look sharp.
Spend money on yourself. Feel good about yourself. Second, focus on the fact that you need
help from your prospective partners in making
a joint decision about whether you should be
together. When they reject you, they're helping
you make the best decision. If you feel physically attracted to someone, you may need his or
her help. Third, be proactive and put yourself in
a position where you're meeting lots of women,
then if you're rejected, pick yourself up and get
back in the race. You'll quickly find that someone new will come along. Fourth, think about
why you're being rejected. At GE, when someone I selected turned me down, I tried to figure
out why, since, obviously, I thought there was a
possibility of a match there, or I wouldn't have
selected that person.

Decisions About Sex

Sooner or later you must make decisions about
sex. The first decision is to wait to have sex.
The right time for finding out about your sexual
compatibility is after you know you match well
on the other 15 differences and when you trust
each other enough to talk openly about the
things that must be discussed. Don't just have
sex decide to have sex.

     Let's begin by saying that sex is one of the

most wonderful things that can happen to you in this material, human world. Under the right circumstances nothing is better. Sex is so good that it ought to be saved for the right time and the right person.

It's true that our hormones drive us to have sex before our emotions have caught up, but we don't have to act on our impulse. The problem with acting on impulse and having sex early in the relationship is that you deepen your attachment to someone that may not be very well matched on the other differences. At that point, the two options you have are equally painful. Stay in the wrong relationship with the wrong partner and spend the rest of your life making it work – or rather making your relationship limp along – or ending the relationship. Rejection is that much more painful when you've become accustomed to someone and have slept with them.

Potential consequences of sexual activity are so devastating – pregnancy at the wrong time and with the wrong partner or sexually transmitted diseases that may kill you – that you must exercise your wisdom and restraint and wait. Decide to have sex at the right time and with the right partner.

Don't have sex until you're certain that your partner will maintain exclusivity in your relationship. That means that neither of you will have sexual relations with anyone else.

Decide on a method of birth control to prevent pregnancy mutually. You are not ready to have a sexual relationship with someone until you can talk about having adult, responsible sex. A birth control method exists for everyone. Information is available from your doctor, a doctor or midwife specializing in the practice of reproductive medicine, or Planned Parenthood.

To have safe sex – primarily to make certain you will not be exposed to HIV and the potential to contract AIDS – use a condom for the first six months of a new sexual relationship. Both partners should be tested for HIV prior to the initiation of a sexual relationship and again at six months. Do not have unprotected sex with your partner unless you can be certain that neither partner has had any other partner during the six-month period and unless both of you test negative for HIV. Certainty about your safety can only occur when you have absolute trust in each other.

Should You Wait For Sex Until Marriage?

Sex is so personal and special that we believe in the idea of saving yourself for marriage, but in practice, waiting until marriage for sex is a huge risk.

We believe that you should wait to have sex until you are all but certain that you've found your perfect partner. That means knowing that you match on the other 15 differences that make a difference.

The reason we advocate beginning a sexual relationship after you're reasonably certain that you've found the right partner, but before marriage is that you must know about your sexual compatibility. Sex is far too important to leave to chance. The key is to act responsibly. When you limit your sexual activity to someone that you have every reason to believe is your perfect partner you act responsibly. When you practice safe sex and use birth control, you act responsibly.

Remember that marriage is for adults. That means sex is for adults.

Sexual Skill

Just like everything else in life, when you're competent you perform more effectively. Sex is no exception. Great sex is a component of a great marriage and so important that we've devoted an entire chapter to great sex, but we want to touch briefly on sexual skill here, as part of basic adult dating skill.

To have good sex you must know what you're doing. Men don't have much trouble with arousal and sexual satisfaction. They become easily aroused, they're best stimulated by the act of intercourse. Sex for men if fairly straightforward. Not so for women. Both men and women have similarities and differences in their sexual function, but women have far more variation than men do. Both men and women need to learn about basic human sexual function and they need to know that even if they learn to have good sex with one partner they will still need to fine tune their performance to a new partner.

Men, the majority of women cannot have an orgasm from intercourse. (See our chapter on Great Sex.) Reports of what percentage of women can and cannot have an orgasm from intercourse vary widely, but one thing is for certain. So many cannot, that you must find out what your partner needs and wants you to do for her to have an orgasm. Women that are not consistently sexually satisfied lose interest in sex and become dissatisfied with their relationship and angry and bitter. Of course, they bear the responsibility to let you know what to do, which takes maturity. But you, as men, must be willing to learn about your partner. Do not assume because you've learned the basics that you know what to do for your partner. Ask. In the comfort of emotional safety and a trusting relationship, ask.

He Said

Carolyn and I had sex fairly soon — within six weeks of knowing each other. I felt that this was fairly fast since I was looking for a long-term partner and not just trying to get laid. I worried about getting a disease. What would I do if I caught something and then had to tell the person whom I had finally found as a long-term partner that I had it, and that she was going to get it too? What a nightmare!

So, why did we have sex so fast? First of all, since we met through Great Expectations, we knew a great deal about each other. We'd read each other's profiles and looked at our videos. Second, I had been dating, and working at finding a long-term partner for a year and nine months. Because I'd been shopping around, having dated or been around many, many women, and I knew what I was looking for, when I finally found it, it was clear to me quickly. Third, before our first date, we had three long phone conversations where we both voluntarily disclosed a tremendous amount of information. I felt that the more she knew about me the better. When I was dating, I always tried to disclose as much information about myself as possible. I didn't want some unpleasant surprise to surface down the road. I had learned from my first marriage just how bad the wrong marriage can be. The net result of all of this was that we were able to exchange a lot of information quickly; and going to bed when it happened was the next logical step in finding out how we'd be together.

I have to tell you that I didn't follow my own rules all of the time about when to have sex, and here's an example of what happened to me. I went to a party sponsored by GE, and I met a successful, attractive woman who was four years older than I was. The room we were partying in had a dance floor, and over on the side, some comfortable, private sofas. We danced and talked in private. It was very romantic. I asked her out. We went into Baltimore the next Sunday, and then I asked her back to my place.

We decided to watch TV on a queen size futon on the floor. We started to kiss and make-out and suddenly she became extremely passionate, lying on top of me kissing me furiously. So now, in the extraordinary heat of passion, we both came up against the problem of birth control and protection from disease. She asked, almost desperately, if I had any condoms. I didn't. I hate the way they feel, covering up the most sensitive parts of my penis to the point where it's hard to maintain an erection for me, anyway. I had decided not to go to bed with anyone where I would need a condom, but here I was naked in bed with this extraordinarily passionate woman. My penis couldn't take the emotional overload of having to think about disease and birth control, and it went up for a short time, and then went down to half-mast.

I still remember some important thoughts and feelings about this affair. I believed her when she said that she wanted a rubber because she was afraid of catching something, not because she wanted to protect me from something she had. In retrospect it was foolish on my part to have taken a risk like that. Her figure wasn't terrific, so that I didn't feel strongly attracted to her, in spite of the fact that I respected and admired her. I felt flattered by the fact that she had such a strong attraction to me, and I told her so. But I also told her that I didn't think things would work out between us. Big mistake! This hurt her feelings quite a bit, and unleashed a torrent of emotions focused at me. I felt deeply troubled by how upset she was. I wished that I hadn't been so impulsive and had sex with her so soon.

And then, about ten days later, I got a small sore on my penis. I was horrified that I might have syphilis or something else. I called her and we talked about it, and she convinced me that it wasn't her. I got the flu about this time, and I had the doctor check me out and take a syphilis test at the same time. I was OK, but it scared me badly.

Later, I continued to have decisions to make about sex.

I went on a sailing trip with the ski club across the Chesapeake Bay. We moored at a marina, went swimming in the pool, and used their facilities. In the evening we went into town to have dinner as a group, and after dinner I found myself walking home alone with a tall, dark-haired, attractive female engineer named Nancy. She was nice, and I was physically attracted to her to some extent, but I knew that we weren't right for each other, because she had a tendency to talk all the time among other things. I'd never get a word in edgewise. She was still tangled up with her ex-husband, and in fact, they got back together some months later, but at this moment in time she was available. I thought that, after we got back to the boats, I could get a blanket and go over along the beach for some serious making-out.

What should I do? Obviously if I lay down under the stars with her, things could easily go too far. What kind of emotional fallout would there be if we went to bed one time and then I had to meet her at every other ski club activity that I went on? The simple answer is that since she didn't fit my long-term goals (and I was fairly certain of this because I knew her from other ski club activities), I shouldn't go any further with her. On the other hand, what could be wrong with a night under the stars, making love?

I decided not to do anything, and after a wonderful walk back to the boats we split up. But when I got back to my boat, there was another woman there! She was with the boat next to mine. I'd helped her out one time by giving her a spare bike tube when hers had gone flat. She asked me, seductively, if there was anything she could do to repay me for my kindness. I was sorely tempted by the thoughts of another fairly attractive woman, under a blanket, under the stars, and naked with me. Twice in one night. Wow!

I decided not to do anything. The truth of the matter is that, at that point, I was strongly committed to my plan to find a long-term partner. My physical attraction to either one of these women wasn't enough to overpower either my determination to stick to my plan or my fear of the downside risks of something bad happening. But these kinds of situations are a common risk of dating. It's easy to be so strongly attracted physically to someone that you get carried away, even though you know they're not right for you.

This story also illustrates some good techniques to attract women. By this time in my dating career I was pretty self-confident. I'd been out with a fair number of women. I'd been working on my packaging. I was in good physical condition, and I had good clothes. The result was that I was attracting women as I went on activities that I was enjoying. I was sizing up quite a few women without actually dating them. But there's a major disadvantage to this approach compared with a dating service like

GE: It's still tough to approach someone who interests you at a ski club function, and it's much easier through a dating service like GE to find out about people.

We recommend you wait to have sex. Treat your sexual expression with the respect it deserves.

8

Choosing to Fall In Love

Five Crucial Questions

alling in love is a decision, not a tidal wave of emotion that sweeps away all sensibility. In fact, love is a verb not an emotion. Love is behavior, over which you have control. You choose to love someone.

We know this is a new idea for most of you, as are some of the other ideas we have. But stop and think about this for a moment. Most people confuse feelings of affection, sexual attraction, sexual desire, admiration, friendliness, compassion, and warmth, with love. Many people confuse feelings of fear, loneliness, neediness, and desperation with love. None of those feelings is love.

Love is the way you treat someone. Love is relating to someone openly and honestly and respectfully. Love is relating to others from a win-win perspective. Love is teaching your children manners and competence. Love is when you take care of yourself because you like yourself and others are depending on you. Love is when you regard the welfare of your partner or your child on par with your own. Love is interdependence. Love is being all that you can be. Love is being sensitive to other's needs and balancing their needs with your own. Love is walking away from the new attraction you feel toward someone because you've made a commitment to another person. The most loving thing you can do for another is to be your real self. Love is not expecting others to take you the way you are if that's less than you can be or if you're obnoxious and demanding or self-centered – of course, unless you're a child and you haven't yet outgrown your natural egocentricity. Children get to be self-centered and demanding – that's part of being a child. Adults don't. Children outgrow those qualities as they experience life and have loving behavior modeled for them by others. Children outgrow egocentricity by getting their needs met as children. Love is not taking others for granted. Love is not hiding your true thoughts and feelings. Love is not accommodating to others so they'll like you or so you won't rock the boat. Love is not convenience.

"Love means never having to say you're sorry," is hogwash.

These lists are by no means complete. But you get the idea. Perfect partners are capable of adult love.

Because love is behavior you can choose to love. You can choose whom to give your long-term loyalty to. The key is to select someone for marriage that giving your love to comes naturally, not someone that asks you to love despite every mismatch and challenge to your integrity.

Pragmatism Does Not Preclude Romance

When you find the right partner, choosing to fall in love is simply happiness and joy without the emotional roller coaster ride. Unfortunately, many of us mistake the excitement and turmoil of a mismatched relationship for love – and the stability of a great relationship for boredom. To help you avoid these mistakes, to help you know whether your partner is capable of adult love and being your perfect partner, we ask you five crucial questions that will enable you to decide about whether you and your partner have the potential for a great marriage. These five questions give you the information you need to decide whether to fall in love.

Five Crucial Questions

1. 16 Differences That Make a Difference – Do you match?
2. How effective is the person?
3. Does this person have his or her head straight?

4. Is your partner genuine, honest, and trust-worthy? Do they have character and integrity?
5. Is there some magic? Are you attracted to each other?

Because love is a decision, you can decide not to fall in love until the time is right.

Question 1: 16 Differences That Make a Difference – Do you match?

You must score your partner and you on each of the 16 differences that make a difference. Review each of the differences and rate your degree of match from one (least match) to 10 (most match). Add your scores for all 16 differences.

If your score is:

Less than 80	Don't even consider this a good match
81-130	You are settling for less than the best
131-160	This is the range where you have the best chance to have a great marriage

One more vital point: You cannot have any very low scores. If you score 0-4 on any single difference you'd better think twice. And if you have more than one very low score you should think seriously of moving on.

Question 2: How effective is the person?

By effective we mean effective as Stephen Covey defines effective in The Seven Habits of Highly Effective People.

Effective people:
-Are able to define what is truly important
-Are able to accomplish worthwhile goals
-Lead rich, rewarding, and balanced lives

Ineffective people:
-Have too much to do in too little time
-Are busy doing mostly unimportant things
-May succeed in one area of life and fail in other areas
-Feel out of control of their lives
-Feel like all they ever do is manage crises
-Don't get what they want out of life
-Don't feel excited about their life
-Don't grow
-Aren't peaceful
-Don't have a sense of meaning or purpose in life

A great marriage is built of two equal partners that are each adequate and competent. They think for themselves and their actions are based on conscious direction. They can each handle the tasks of daily living.

Each partner was normally dependent to varying degrees during their childhood, gradually out-growing the child's self-centeredness and inexperience, to become evermore able to relate to others in an emotionally healthy way and evermore competent. By outgrowing dependence by living through it and mastering competence – rather than skipping it and pretending to be competent and mature when not in reality, each partner reaches the independence required to function at their best in the adult world.

However, independence is not the ultimate goal. Rather, interdependence is the mode of relatedness that comes from maturity. No man is an island. All of us live better when we can collaborate with others. The most competent and adequate person still needs others at times.

The mode of relatedness you are seeking in an effective partner is the ability to function interdependently. That means you will each be able to competently handle the tasks of daily living. And it means that during times of high stress or illness that you can each lean on the other, temporarily. You are neither diminished nor crippled by temporary leaning or being leaned upon.

A great marriage doesn't just mean making it through the day. A great marriage means soaring through the day.

Ask yourself

What does your partner say is important in life? Do they have a good job that they are happy doing? What goals has your partner accomplished and what goals does he or she have for the future? What in his or her life makes your partner lead a rich, rewarding, and balanced life? How well does your partner handle the tasks of daily living? Do they go to work regularly? Do they pay their bills on time? Do they live within their means? Do they feed themselves nourishing meals? Do they keep themselves healthy and fit? Do they keep their clothes clean and in good repair? Do they avoid addictive habits? Do they keep their car and home in good repair? Do they keep their living environment clean and orderly?

Does your partner

Have too much to do in too little time most of the time? Does your partner spend most of his or her time doing tasks that seem trivial – like lots of busywork? Succeed in one area of life and fail in other areas? Feel out of control of his or her life? Feel like all they ever do is manage crises? Get what they want out of life, consistently? Feel excited about his or her life? Demonstrate an effort to stretch and grow psychologically and intellectual? Experience peace? Have a sense of meaning or purpose in life?

A "yes" answer to the first 5 questions and a "no" answer to the last 5 questions show ineffectiveness.

If your partner is marrying age and is ineffective, ask yourself why he or she isn't very effective. Ask yourself if you want to be parental in your relationship to them. Do they show signs of improving their effectiveness? How?

Our opinion is, anyone can improve their effectiveness given some effort and determination, but you're taking a gamble on something that hasn't happened yet and you cannot count on your partner changing. You should make your decision based on the here and now. If you are effective, he or she will not be your equal. He or she won't be a perfect partner contributing to a great marriage.

Remember, marriage is for adults and when you bring yourself to the dating marketplace you need to be all of the things you want your partner to be. Your partner needs to be all they want you to be. If you marry someone that's ineffective you'll spend at least some of your time in a parental role and picking up the slack – or even worse – living a chaotic life.

If your partner is somewhat effective, you have a better chance, but all of the same applies. People do continue to mature. If they don't, you may be able to live with the amount of ineffectiveness they bring into your life, depending on how ineffective he or she is.

When you and your partner are highly effective, you have the makings of a great marriage with a high level of satisfaction. You can have a marriage where you will both contribute to the best you each can be and to the best a marriage can be.

Question 3: Does your partner have his or her head straight?

Remember that getting your head straight means knowing who you are, matching your behavior to who you are, and liking yourself.

The way you feel about yourself influences how you relate to every person and situation in your life. The way you feel about yourself affects how you think about and interpret events. The way you understand events in your environment filters through the way you feel about yourself. When you feel good about yourself you convey to others that you believe in yourself. When you feel good about yourself, getting others to believe in you is relatively easy. When you feel good about yourself you expect that good will happen to you. Your expectation of happy endings results in happy endings.

People that don't know themselves attune their behaviors to what others expect and they behave as extensions of others from whom they seek approval. They count what others think about what's important more than they count what they think about what's important. When you don't know whom you are how can you know with whom you should match on the 16 differences? How can you be effective?

If you know who you are, but act like someone else, what difference does it make that you know who you are? Acting like someone other than who you are will get you a life other than what you want and other than what's good for you. If you accommodate to others, think about the layers of resentment that will build over time. Can you live, or even like someone for whom you feel so much resentment? Can you be effective when your actions reflect someone else's beliefs rather than your own? How can someone that molds their behaviors to others' opinions have control over his or her life? The most ironic thing of all is that, people that don't have control over their own life try to control everyone else's life. They do that to have a measure of predictability over their life, but it doesn't work.

And not only do you have to know yourself and behave like yourself, you must like yourself. How can someone else like you if you don't like you? People with healthy ways of thinking become cautious about those that transmit signals that you should be cautious about them. People with healthy ways of thinking, effective people, don't want to slow themselves down to carry the load of someone that should be carrying their own load. How would you feel about yourself if you knew you were slowing others down? That would add to your not feeling good about yourself or thinking admirably about yourself. When there is something about yourself that you don't like, change it. First, think about whether the quality deserves to have you disapprove or whether it's a quality that's fine, but that someone else has told you is bad. Think for yourself. Is the quality really bad? If it is, change it. If it isn't then stop feeling bad about it.

But liking yourself isn't arrogance. We

need to make sure you can distinguish between people who genuinely like themselves and someone who has an inflated sense of self or arrogance.

People that like themselves:
- Don't have any need to control and manipulate others
- Quietly go about making their lives happy and satisfying
- Attract people that like them, too
- Attract positive experiences
- Have certain limits and boundaries
- Rarely have crises to manage
- Like to learn about others' ideas and beliefs
- Can relate to many different kinds of people
- Toot their own horn in a dignified way
- Are realistic about their strengths and limitations
- Don't waste their time trying to be all things to all people
- May critique the behavior and opinions of others just to think ideas through for themselves, but don't have a need to make others into their own image
- Choose how to spend their time and with whom
- Make the most out of what they have
- Take responsibility for their lives, acting in accordance with their values
- Are fit and healthy
- Choose healthy relationships in which to be involved

People that don't like themselves:
   -Use a variety of active and passive behaviors
     to manipulate and control others
   -Attract people that don't like them
   -Often defend an inner sense of inferiority
     with an air of superiority
   -Feel humiliated by being less than perfect
   -Fear and abhor any kind of criticism, includ-
     ing constructive criticism
   -Criticize others, as well as themselves
   -Have a low tolerance for mistakes
   -Rarely take chances or try new things
   -Are self-effacing
   -Have low self-acceptance
   -Depend on the opinion of others for their
     self-esteem; approval bolsters self-esteem
     (or pseudo self-esteem) temporarily; disap-
     proval sends their self-esteem crashing to
     the bottom of the pit
   -Sometimes have an inflated sense of what
     they can do and can't allow themselves to
     know what they don't know

   The lists could go on, but you get the
idea. Arrogance is the opposite of healthy self-
esteem. In many cases superiority is a façade
and demonstrates inferiority through the behavior of someone that thinks and acts as though
they're better than others are. Of course, some
people truly believe that they are better than
others are. Someone that likes himself or herself is humble, but realistic about whom they
are.
   All of these ideas apply to your prospective partner. Get your own head straight and

then make sure your partner has his or her head straight.

Question 4: Is your partner genuine, honest, and trustworthy? Do they have character and integrity?

One reason why this question is so important is that many marriages break up because of infidelity. You need to know whether your partner is likely to cheat on you. Whether infidelity happens because your partner is unhappy due to incompatibility or whether it happens because your partner lacks the ability to keep his or her commitment is a moot point. Infidelity hurts not matter what its reason.

No one believes that infidelity can happen to them, but according to one recent survey 70 percent of all men commit adultery. You can use that statistic to support the notion that men are just not monogamous creatures, but the fact that 30 percent are loyal says otherwise. We believe that if women would refuse to have relationships with and marry disloyal men,

The qualities that we will discuss here are necessary for a high level of adult function; the level of function that a great marriage requires.

Genuineness

Someone who is genuine tells you who he or she really is with his or her words and behavior.

Their talk and deeds are filled with sincerity and match. They don't put on airs. They don't wear masks. They're not phony. They don't hide themselves from you. When they tell you how they feel you can believe them. Being genuine means living honestly. They don't say they aren't angry with you with clenched fists and jaw. They don't con you with empty compliments. They don't charm you just to get their way.

Your perfect partner is genuine.

Honesty

Honest people tell the truth and live the truth. Some people are dishonest unintentionally and some people are dishonest intentionally. Neither can have a great marriage. Honest people are worthy of trust. Dishonest people, whether dishonest intentionally or unintentionally, cannot be trusted.

Your perfect partner is honest.

Trustworthy

Have you ever been blamed for not trusting others? Some people believe that there is something wrong with someone that doesn't trust someone else. It's true that some people have been harmed psychologically and have difficulty trusting others even if they may be worthy of trust. With some work with trustworthy people these people can repair their inability to trust.

But most people have the capacity to trust others. When those people don't trust someone it's important for them to listen to themselves so something bad doesn't happen to them.

The point that those people who accuse you or others of not trusting them or someone else misses is that someone must be worthy of trust if you are to trust them. Isn't it terribly foolish to trust someone that isn't worthy of trust just to give them the benefit of the doubt?

On the other hand, sometimes when a person cannot trust others they are projecting onto the other person. What that means is that since they themselves cannot be trusted they believe that no one else can be trusted.

In any case, you must pay attention and live through enough experiences with someone to determine whether or not they are worthy of trust. And you should make a conscious decision about whether to trust someone not blindly trust others.

You can trust perfect partners and they can trust you.

Character

A person with character has moral and ethical strength. J.C. Watts, Rep. from Oklahoma, says, "character is doing what's right when no one is looking." Living by guiding principles helps us do what is right and helps us respect others and ourselves.

Developing a conscience assists with moral and ethical strength. Many people do what's right because they're afraid they'll get caught. People with character do what's right just because it feels better – they like themselves when they do what's right.

Your perfect partner has character.

Integrity

Someone with integrity lives up to his or her principles and values. They don't compromise and negotiate something they believe is right or wrong. Someone with integrity doesn't abandon their values and principles because someone else teases them or disapproves of them. They don't say one thing and do another.

Perfect partners have integrity.

Each one of these qualities works with the others. It's difficult to separate them, but each also has subtle aspects of its own. Your partner having or not having these qualities can mean the difference between a poor marriage, a marriage of convenience, and a great marriage. Partners having these qualities add more positive energy to your relationship. When your partner has these qualities, you won't have to spend your time and energy on managing crises, losses, and emotional pain as a regular part of your relationship.

Perfect partners are genuine, honest, trustworthy, and they have character and integrity.

Question 5: Is there some magic? Are you attracted to each other?

Most people base their belief that they've found the right partner on chemistry and physical attraction. They believe that if you have plenty of chemistry it must mean love.

That's wrong. Physical attraction – chemistry – is important, but you can't make it the first and only thing on which you base your selection. That is, if you want a great marriage rather than a poor marriage or a marriage of convenience, you can't base your choice of partner just on magic.

We've deliberately made this question last because only having magic isn't enough and too many people believe that it's the primary factor. Being physically attracted is the icing on the cake not the cake. If you can't answer the four previous questions affirmatively, no matter how much chemistry you have you'll never have a great marriage. You'll have another one of those marriages that you'll have to work very hard at to make work.

You can and will be attracted to many more people in this world than your partner. Noticing the attraction makes us feel good, but making a commitment to our partner means not following though on the attraction. And being attracted doesn't mean you match on the 16 differences or that the other three questions have affirmative answers.

On the other hand, someone with whom you match very well and you can answer the three other questions in the affirmative can build some magic with you over time that just gets stronger and stronger as time goes by.

If everything else looks good for this to be your perfect partner, then if you have some excitement to begin with – even at the level of looking forward to having a fun and interesting time with them – the chances are that magic will follow quickly behind. Feeling instant intense physical attraction is far more likely to blind you to other problems in the relationship than to indicate that you've found your perfect partner.

Doesn't it make sense to you that spending time with someone that's interesting and mature and that has compatible values can develop an intensifying attraction as you build a history together? Magic with the right partner deepens and intensifies over time. Your attunement and the supportive climate for being who you really are sparks magic, electricity, and energy. Magic with the wrong partner can leave as suddenly as it came.

After You've Decided to Fall in Love, Help Them Fall in Love With You

When the conditions are right, you can help your perfect partner fall in love with you. This is where mature charm and seduction are useful. Romantic things like sending flowers, calling every day, sending cards, flirting, or many other things that you know your partner appreciates will inspire falling in love. Your increasing togetherness will begin to create a history together: Little things that are private between the two of you that will continue to cement the bond.

Good relationship skills will allow constructive communication. Constructive communication will increase the emotional safety of your relationship. The rush of new love excitement will create the bond; the history building together will extend the excitement into long-term love with loyalty, appreciation, affection, and continued growth.

How do you get someone who you want to fall in love with you?

Lisa, while in therapy with Carolyn, told the story of her falling in love with her perfect partner over the weeks. She'd come into therapy when a 10-year live-in relationship ended and she was grieving. For several weeks she worked through issues from that relationship and gradually gained some perspective. She came to see what she really wanted. As she resolved her grief she was able to get to know herself better than she ever had and was able to define what she wanted and the kind of person that could be her perfect partner.

Meanwhile, she'd been getting to know someone knew as a friend. She enjoyed talking to Bob; they had a lot in common. They found talking to each other to be fun and interesting. After several weeks and when Bob sensed that Lisa was open to dating him, he asked her out. They dated a few times and gradually explored the idea of having a romantic relationship with the possibility of marriage in the future.

Initially Lisa felt scared but excited. They began to increase their intimacy. Lisa felt skittish and a few times seemed to sabotage their increasing closeness. Fortunately, with the help of therapy, she could see what she was doing and began to work on her fear of intimacy. Carolyn helped Lisa explore her past, including her parents' marriage, for established patterns. She could see that some of her behaviors in male-female relationships were a habit she'd developed left over from her mother's behavior with her father. Choosing consciously not to act that way anymore helped Lisa learn more constructive behavior and helped her overcome a habit of relating that ruined her relationships.

Using the five crucial questions, Lisa was able to be objective about what to know about Bob and their relationship. Having an objective perspective gave Lisa the stability and confidence to proceed. Bob persisted even when things got a bit shaky. And in the end, Bob got just what he wanted. Lisa found her perfect partner and decided she wanted to marry Bob.

He said

How to get someone to fall in love with you is a question as old and as important as life itself. When I think back on how I got Carolyn to fall in love with me, I realized, much to my surprise, that I actually used many of the techniques that great salesmen use when they're selling a fine product. As much as our culture romanticizes falling in loving, I believe that the same types of factors that influence them when they buy a product heavily influence most people in their decisions. For example, I was serious about one woman I dated, named Doris, who made about $65,000 per year (which was more than I was making at the time) and had made up to $85,000 per year. When we were discussing how well we might fit together as long-term partners, she told me, rather bluntly, that I was a middle-aged employee of a company that could go under. She'd decided not to fall in love with me because I didn't make as much money as she wanted.

When I first met Carolyn, I talked freely and honestly about myself. I wanted to disclose as much information about myself as possible because I wanted to know how well we matched, and I needed her help to figure that out. I wanted to build trust. If she was going to believe what I'd be saying to her in the future and how our lives could be together, then it was vital that she trust me. One of the reasons why some people become so guarded in their contacts with the opposite sex is that they've met so many slick and dishonest people out in the dating marketplace (or should I say the dating jungle). Being honest and building trust is an extremely effective technique to overcome this barrier.

There's a form of dishonesty that has ruined many long-term relationships. When people first start dating, they want the other person to like them, and so they're accommodating. After they're married they reveal their true self; they're no longer accommodating, and the relationship breaks up. I dated one woman who was so accommodating that I could hardly stand it. I wanted to find out what she was really like, and I couldn't. Carolyn was honest and straightforward with me right from the beginning.

I began selling myself to Carolyn before I ever met her. I did it with marketing help from GE. They helped me advertise myself. They helped me tell other people how valuable I was. In doing my profile and video, I also had help from the most important person of all – myself! I had help from myself because I believed in myself. I believed there was someone out there just right for me and that I would be a wonderful gift to them. Now, I'm not saying there weren't periods when I had serious self-doubts. There were. But I believed in what I was selling – me. You've all had experiences where you've bought fine products from good sales persons. You could tell they believed in what they were selling. It makes a tremendous difference. It's one of the reasons we've put so much emphasis in this book on getting your head straight.

I was persistent in my pursuit of women in general and Carolyn in particular. This is another characteristic of good sales people. When I asked women out, I wouldn't take no for an answer until the third time. On two occasions I actually went over to see women who had turned me down for a second date.

Four reasons why persistence pays:

1. The number of people who match you is small. In sales terms, you have to

make a lot of calls to make a sale.

2. People are often guarded because they're afraid of the negative emotional overhead that often goes with dating. They may disguise their true feelings, seeming to be totally uninterested when they are interested but are afraid of the risks of getting involved. They don't want to show that they're interested. It takes time and persistence to get past this barrier.

3. People may have children, parents, or friends who are giving them advice or rules on whom to be with. For example, Carolyn's mother thought, based on my profile, that I was right for her. This almost finished me off, because Carolyn didn't want her mother telling her what to do. Carolyn was dating someone else when I first called her, and she almost didn't go out with me because one of her rules was that she shouldn't be dating more than one person at a time. Fortunately, some other friends convinced her that it was a good idea to shop around.

4. Timing can be critical in dating. People often need time to get used to you and to make up their minds and to think about you. When people don't know what they want or who they are, making big decisions can be tough, and they need time to work things through. Being persistent means being patient, waiting for them to date other people if

necessary.

On our first date we went out to dinner
and to a movie: a typical first date. This first
date was remarkable, however. By this time I'd
been on enough first dates to know that the
same topics tend to come up over and over
again. Where do you live? What's your job like?
Why'd you break up with your ex-wife? What
are your kids like? I tried to cover every one of
these first date questions on the phone before
we went out. As part of my plan to sell myself to
Carolyn, I wanted her to have a good time with
me. One of the things I was selling was that she
was going to have fun with me. Our life together would be good. When we went out on that
first date, we had a great time. I got Carolyn
involved in the product, me, in a positive way.

After we'd been out several times, I began
to think hard about how well we fit together and
whether we were right for each other. I thought
we matched extremely well. We had a long
phone conversation during which I talked about
what our life would be like together. I talked
about how we could travel and have fun together. I told her about my kids and the financial
commitment I had to them; but I emphasized
that we'd do well together financially. I knew
enough about her from the questions that I'd
asked to know that we both wanted the same
things. The next Sunday, after this phone call, I
went out on a hiking trip I'd planned with the
ski club. When I got back, I came over to see
Carolyn, and she did some selling herself. She
showed me around her house. It was neat in

some places, but not so neat in others. I felt right at home. We cuddled and kissed, listened to music, and talked the night away in front of the fireplace.

When I talked to Carolyn the next day, she told me that she couldn't get to sleep last night because she was thinking about me. Wow! Fantastic! I knew I was golden. I was still concerned about sex. I'd had so much trouble with sex in the past that I was worried about it. But I had extraordinarily strong feelings that this was the moment in my life when I was finally going to find the right partner. It was a turning point. Everything in my life that followed from here on out was remarkably different.

I ordered flowers to be delivered the next day. I put a message with the flowers: "You are the one that I have been looking for all of my life! Love, Wes." When the flowers arrived at the hospital where Carolyn worked, her knees got shaky. It was a wonderful moment for her to share with the people with whom she worked. They all knew her story, and how her husband had passed away.

About four o'clock that day, I called her at work to talk to her. Over the phone, in a throaty voice, I said that she was the one that I'd been looking for all of my life. I asked her if she wanted to go to Williamsburg, Virginia for the weekend with me. She said yes. I wanted to go to Williamsburg because I felt that this would bond us. It was also an indirect way of bringing up sex, since it was obvious to both of us that if we were going away for the weekend we'd be sleeping together. I wanted to know how sex would be for us. I wanted us to be together so that she would learn more about me and value me. It was part of my selling myself to her.

On Wednesday I came over to Carolyn's house. We watched TV in the family room. We'd now arrived at the moment where sex was the issue at hand. I was nervous. I told Carolyn that I'd had trouble with impotence in the past. I told her about my problems with sex with my ex-wife. Here's where Carolyn did a wonderful job selling herself by partnering with me to create great sex. She listened to me. I felt accepted and loved. Everything was going to be OK. She said that, since she had her period, there was no need to rush. This took a lot of the pressure to perform off of me. So, that night we basically just explored each other.

On Friday we went to Williamsburg. We made love twice a day for four days. Carolyn had multiple orgasms. I can still remember how proud and happy I was on Saturday.

We had a wonderful time at Williamsburg. We walked, talked, and saw the sights. We went out to dinner.

Our last day in Williamsburg over brunch, the question of marriage came up in a casual way. I suggested moving in together because I didn't want to be apart after such a wonderful time together. Carolyn said that we could save money on taxes if we were married, which, of course, isn't true anymore. So I said that my goal was to be married again. When we got back home, I got enough of my belongings to begin moving in together. The next night, after thinking about the whole thing, and after we teased again about taxes and marriage, I agreed that we should go ahead and get married. And Carolyn said "yes", she'd like that. I didn't consider my proposal of marriage a big deal because, as far as I was concerned, we were already married. We were going to spend the rest of our lives together. However, I did feel it was important for everyone to know we were married, so I agreed happily to a formal ceremony.

All of this romancing didn't take long, less than six weeks. We announced the marriage to my relatives at Thanksgiving dinner. Everyone was surprised, to say the least.

Understand – the issue is when you have enough information about someone to answer the five crucial questions, not the number of weeks or months you've known someone.

Commitment!

Why is it the woman's job to hook and land a man? Because commitment or fear of commitment is almost always a man's issue, it's useful to explore some of the things we think contribute to his reluctance to commit and what we think you can do.

One theory is the idea that men have a basic instinct – a biological, animal instinct – to impregnate as many women as possible to assure the advancement of the species and contribute to the gene pool. Maybe, maybe not. Animal species do exist that spread their seed around. The only problem with that explanation is that we, as humans, have a cortex in our brain that allows for thinking. The cortex allows us to be proactive (think about what to do between stimulus and response). That makes us different from other animals. We also have advantages to making family units in which to raise our young. And, in fact, there are animal species that mate for life, and many men who have no desire to stray.

Given that humans can think, the advantages to having family units, and the fact that some animal species mate for life, isn't it possible that what gets in the way of men making commitments may stem from something else? Maybe this animal/biology business is just an excuse used to explain something more threatening to the image we have of ourselves!

What if there's another explanation? Would understanding another angle help men and women deal with this issue?

We think many men have difficulty with intimacy due to what they think it means to be a man. Imagine being told, probably by age 5, that to cry when you're hurt, or to run home to the safety of mom, meant you were a sissy or a mommy's boy! You spent your childhood trying your best not to be either. Suddenly you become a young man, attracted to women romantically and sexually. Of course, during your childhood, even though you did your best to bury your desires for your mother's comfort, you continued to want and need the reassurance of her presence and help. This sets up a tremendous necessity to deny a basic need – that of self-disclosure to a caring individual. OOPS! There's the forerunner for intimacy! If society did its job well, here you are a man and every time you attempt to get emotionally close to a woman it triggers deep anxiety. It challenges your idea of what it takes to be a man! And the chances are that what happened to make you feel so threatened by warmth, tenderness, and intimacy, happened so long ago you don't even remember how you came to believe what it takes to be a man. Suddenly, here you are trying to establish your skills at mating, and every time you get close you go into a tailspin!

Commitment is a major issue for many men, particularly men who were raised before the 70s. It still goes on, but men are currently freer to feel all of their feelings and turn to their mom for support. If this is an issue for you, it'll take courage, time, and effort on your part to unravel how it came to be an issue, and to grieve having missed early opportunities to practice intimacy. If this is an issue for you, only then will you be able to overcome your fears and re-establish the ability to be intimate.

Now, in all fairness! There could be another side to the commitment issue some of the time. Women are likewise raised with certain rules and expectations; they often grow up unable to be their true selves. They lose touch with what they believe. They learn to deny what they see and hear, loosing touch with their feelings. The outcome of this contributes to women disguising themselves and learning to accommodate others' wants and needs. In doing so they give up who they are.

When a woman gives up who she is, it deprives her of a real life, and it deprives both of information about how well they match. It doesn't take many relationships where the woman has disguised her real self, accommodated to the man, only to show her true self later, to make a man gun shy! Let's say you're a man who believes you match well with a woman on the differences that make a difference. You don't realize she isn't being truthful about who she is, and make a commitment to her. If you then learned what a terrible mistake this relationship was only after you'd gotten married, wouldn't you be afraid of commitment too?

The point is fear of commitment isn't something to use as an excuse to never commit. It's merely more information about yourself that you can choose to unravel and ultimately use to your advantage. Are you afraid to commit not only to this person, but also to others? Use your answer to begin to understand how you came to be afraid. Would you like to know yourself better so you can find your perfect partner? Once again, if you've done your ground work, gotten your head straight, and identified who you are, you'll more than likely be able to overcome any reluctance to commit. You can find your perfect partner by following our suggestions.

She said

An issue came up for my son one day when I was talking about this book and marriage. He was hesitating about making a commitment to someone who's well matched to him. In looking back through his issues, we saw that he'd suffered when his father and I divorced, had seen many of his friends' parents divorce, had seen many unhappy marriages, had seen devastating divorces, and had himself been in a miserable marriage a few years ago, which lasted three months. Making the decision to leave that marriage was the most painful thing he'd ever had to do. He'd come to believe that no relationship could make it long-term. He was thinking that maybe people should just live together so it wouldn't be so difficult to leave when the inevitable happened. Listening to my son remember and experience such pain and indecision wasn't the easiest thing I've ever done. But when I thought about his dilemma, this is what I told him:

"It's true that many marriages in the past failed, ending in divorce. Or even worse, miserable marriages that went on and on. Decisions to marry in past generations were based on the need to divide the labor and to have large families to do the work. Many died early, so big families overcame losing the family line. People needed marriages of convenience to survive. They also didn't have much time to be best friends. There wasn't much time for fun and intimacy. It's only been recently that our society has developed the technology to divide the labor differently. Doing so has released us to have time for other activities. The nature of relationships and what people want and need from them is changing. It isn't that it's impossible to have a marriage that can last long-term and be wonderful – it's that we don't know how to choose the right partner for that kind of marriage. We haven't had much practice at it, and there aren't many role models to show us how. I asked him to re-think the situation and to consider the possibility that marriages of yesterday didn't last, or weren't the best because we didn't know how to choose our partners. Now we know more, and we have a better chance of choosing the partner that will fit with our new needs. People are evolving. Society is evolving. Needs are evolving. I believe strongly in marriage, and I believe it's possible to choose your partner to encourage marriage's permanence."

Focus on win-win. Remember that you want the relationship to be great for you as well as the other person! Answer the five questions about your prospective partner, making sure you both evaluate how well you match on the sixteen differences. Sit down and talk to each other about the list of attributes answers to the five crucial questions. Don't be mysterious about your answers to each other.

Then – don't drag it on! Make the commitment or get out! If you do match well, but you still have reservations, trust your instinct about it. Listen to yourself. If it doesn't feel right to you, end it! At the same time, if you feel wonderful, feel you match well, and the attraction is there – go for it! As humans were designed to be able to perceive the information we need to make it in life. If you're in touch with your perceptions and listen to what your senses tell you, you won't fail to make accurate decisions!

She said

Falling in love with Wes was easy and wonderful. When I think back over our getting together, I can see we both did some selling. We had a good balance of showing each other just how we felt without going overboard. When he knew that I was beginning to feel attached to him and liked him a lot, he called more often, sent me flowers, and made himself available to me mentally, emotionally, and physically. He made a date with me to go away for the weekend to shift into the next stage of the relationship.

There wasn't one minute where I felt unsure, once I could see how well we matched, how well we got along, and that we were headed in the same direction. Every other relationship I'd been in seemed like a roller coaster ride. I mistook the excitement of the ride for love. This time there was no roller coaster ride, just happiness and peace. I felt excited but secure, not afraid.

Another thing that impressed me about Wes was that he made himself available to being loved. It helps someone to love you when you are lovable and open to being loved.

Part IV

The Great Marriage

9

Great Sex

A Real-Life Example

Caution: Marriage and sex are for adults. Therefore, even though this chapter describes explicit sexual behavior, we believe it is appropriate for any adult that wants to know a variation of great sex. If, for any reason, you feel uncomfortable with such a vivid description of loving, real-life sexual expression, we must caution you to proceed with care or not at all.

We took our time and great care to decide if we would share such personal information with you. Please treat this information with the respect that we also offer it.

The recent survey, <u>Sex In America</u> (Michael, Gagnon, Laumann, and Kolata, 1994), states that measures of sexual satisfaction with primary partners showed:

-75% of men always had an orgasm.

-29% of women always had an orgasm.

-only 46% of men were extremely
 physically pleased.

-only 40% of women were extremely
 physically pleased.

-41% of men said they felt extremely
 emotionally satisfied.

-39% of women said they felt extremely
 emotionally satisfied.

This is truly a sad state of affairs in our estimation.

The Importance of Great Sex

Having great sex:

-will leave you feeling physically satisfied.

-will leave you feeling emotionally
 satisfied.

-will increase trust in your relationship.

-will increase intimacy in your
 relationship.

-helps you stay physically healthy.

-helps you stay emotionally healthy.

-makes your marriage better than a
 marriage of convenience.

-contributes to feeling good about your
 self.

-fosters the kind of climate that facilitates
 reaching your greatest potential.

-fosters the kind of climate that facilitates

your children reaching their greatest vivid description of loving, real-life sexual expression, we must caution you to proceed with care or not at all.

What is Great Sex?

Envision... a beautiful summer evening. The air is fragrant with the perfume of the flowers, and you've just arrived back at your hotel room after a romantic meal with your mate. You've spent the day together; you're well into the first week of your marriage; you're on your honeymoon. Both of you feel full of mental and emotional pleasure, and feel like making love...

Or maybe the two of you have been dating for some time, becoming good friends. You've just spent the day together biking in the cool fall air. You're both invigorated and pleasantly tired. You're filled with fun and laughter from the day, and feel wonderful being together. You've grown to know each other so well that you've discussed things like planning for children, and how you're going to handle any potential sexual risks; and tonight seems like the right time to begin a sexual relationship...

Dream about being on vacation and having spent the morning at Disney World. You've had lunch and taken in a show. You're slowing down after so much activity, and, besides that, it's getting pretty hot in the summer sun. You and your partner head back to your room for some afternoon sex, a nap, and the Jacuzzi, or a swim...

Imagine you wake up on a rainy Sunday morning with the whole day ahead of you. Now that it's raining, you can't do the yard work; so you decide to stay in bed and read the papers. One of you gets the papers from out front, the other fixes some breakfast, and you head back to bed. One thing leads to another and...

Think about you've had a typically difficult day at work. You've been rushing around since 6:30 a.m., have fed and bathed the kids, and put them to bed. Your mate has cleaned up the dinner mess and the two of you head for your bedroom, to read the evening newspapers, or watch the news on TV. After unwinding, the idea of sex sounds like the perfect way to come back to what matters, to renew your connection, and to help you relax to sleep...

Or you awaken to the sound of the alarm (music please), stretch, thinking how nice it would be to stay in bed just a while longer. As you stretch, you feel your partner's body turning and stretching next to yours and, suddenly, all you want is to have sex – just a quickie before work...

Wow! Isn't this as nice as it can be? What all of these scenarios have in common are two people who are good friends, feel terrific about themselves, and have found a partner who matches so well that they rarely have any differences to solve. When they do have differences, they admire and respect each other, they trust each other, and they've developed their communication skills well enough that they're able to find solutions without negative side effects. They're committed to each other in all ways, including dividing the chores in a way acceptable to each. People who are in a relationship with each other this way don't have any difficulty expressing themselves sexually. They have the confidence to know that, whatever their frequency of sex, it's right for them. They feel desirous toward each other often, because they feel good about themselves, about their partner, and about their interactions.

All of this happens apart from sexual technique. Adding to their desire is the knowledge that they've each learned what pleases and satisfies the other.

An Example of How to Have Great Sex

He said

I like sex. And I really like women. Put me in a group of people, when I was single, and you'd find me spending most of my time with the women. When I was in the fifth grade, living in Florida, I got a friend of mine to tell me when his sister was going to take a shower. The shower window had three panes of glass. The lower two were frosted, but the top one wasn't; and after climbing up a tall tree in the back yard, I could see right in. She was beautiful, with a gorgeous black bush of pubic hair. I watched her until she finished taking her shower, and then went around the house where, surprisingly enough, there was a ladder. I climbed up and watched her through her bedroom window, hoping for another look. Unfortunately, I was too distracted to notice one of the neighbors watching. I got off the ladder, went around the house in the other direction, and ran straight into a man with a flashlight, shining it in my face. He asked me some abrupt questions, let me go, and then told my dad the next day. My dad was not happy. He said I should be careful or I might get shot by one of the neighbors. That was the end of that. So much for the budding of young sexual attraction.

I've read a fair amount of literature with a lot of sex in it: Some of it being what most people would call pornography. I've looked at many of the sex books on the market – not pornographic, but designed as self-help – like The Joy of Sex. I've watched X-rated movies, and I've seen many steamy sex scenes in R-rated movies. I've read the Hite report and other books about women having orgasms. What strikes me about all of this sex literature, is that it's still hard to figure out from all of it how to make love to a woman in a way that will leave both partners deeply satisfied and happy. What's missing, I think, are real examples of real people having great sex. People learn best by example. All of the words that you need in order to say anything are in the dictionary. Understanding the words still won't make it possible for you to write a great story. One of the best ways to learn how to write a great story is to read stories other people have written. The same is true of having great sex. When I think about what I know now about how to make a woman feel good, I know I missed some great opportunities in my past to have a wonderful time.

In writing this book, both Carolyn and I asked ourselves how open to be regarding sex. We decided to open up because of the lack of good examples in other literature. We believe so strongly in marriage with the right partner, that we decided to overcome our desire for privacy. Your great relationship isn't all it can be unless there's great sex — for both partners.

Before I start talking about how we go about making love, I want to highlight the point that great sex is the result of a lot of preparation. It's a lot more than just the mechanics, which I'm going to step through in detail shortly. First of all, much of what we talk about in this book can be summed up with the simple statement: You need the right partner. To feel relaxed and ready for sex you can't be in a relationship in which you're working hard to make it work. When you're using your time and energy to negotiate and compromise everything, when your integrity is on the line almost every day, little time, energy, and desire are left for sex and fun. When you spend your lives separate, there's little inspiration to deepen the bond with sexual intimacy. When you're bracing yourself for the next round of differences or name-calling or putdowns, how can you be open and vulnerable enough to expose yourself to a robust sexual relationship?

Great sex is a team effort. It takes good communication and a strong focus on the needs of your partner to find out what your partner likes, and how to make each other feel good. And learning how to make each other feel good, about something so intimate and personal as sex, requires the foundation of a solid relationship.

Second, sex is a physical activity. A man needs a hard penis and good muscles and stamina to control its movement. A hard penis comes from a strong cardiovascular system and from having unclogged blood vessels to the penis. You need strong leg and back muscles to control the motion of your penis during sex. A woman needs strong muscles too, particularly abdominal and pelvic muscles, to have good orgasms. She also needs muscles in order to move her body under the weight of her man or on top of her man. She needs good vaginal muscles to squeeze her man's penis and intensify her own pleasure. This squeezing action clamps down on the base of the penis and pumps the blood up into the head, expanding it and making both partners feel wonderful. Childbirth can stretch vaginal muscles. However, lots of sex and the right exercise program can re-strengthen the muscles in the vagina to the point where a woman can get a powerful grip on her man's penis.

Third, diet can have a big impact on your general heath and, consequently, if you're a man, how hard your penis gets. Speaking as a man, from my personal experience I can tell you that alcohol, nicotine, caffeine, and saturated fat can have a deadly effect on the stiffness of your penis, especially as you get older.

Don't talk to me of love. Show me!

Making love is something that we like to do
every day, sometimes twice a day. In the evening
we start with a transitional period on our big,
firm bed, watching TV and reading the papers. I
say firm bed because I believe that's critical to
good lovemaking. One of the most important
things to me is to control the motion of my
penis when I'm inside Carolyn. A hard bed gives
me a firm platform for my knees to rest on,
which allows me to control the motion of my
penis better. I can't imagine using a waterbed.
Even a slightly softer bed is more work because
I feel that I'm working against the bed.

After a period of unwinding, our minds
begin to switch away from the hassles of the
day. While we're watching TV or reading, I like
to reach over and gently squeeze her clitoris
between my thumb and forefinger, lightly rolling
it like a marble. Or I gently stroke or touch her
breasts. I do this on and off for about fifteen
minutes, then we shut off the TV, push the
papers off the bed, and turn on the radio or CD
player so that we can have soft music in the
background. Carolyn climbs on top of me. We
kiss and talk some more about the day. I cup my
hands on her breasts, squeezing them gently.

After about five to ten minutes of kissing,
hugging, and talking, with her on top of me, we
switch directions, starting what I call the...

Ladies-first phase of lovemaking

Our love-making now focuses exclusively on Carolyn in a series of positions that gradually escalate the level of stimulation and allow me to shift my position a few times so that I don't get tired or bored. One of the good things about having her go first is that I get a chance to relax. The blood has moved out of my limbs and is available to pump up my penis.

But the main reason for Carolyn going first is that she has an orgasm after being stimulated by my tongue and fingers, and then she has multiple orgasms when I enter her with my penis. I call this whole sequence the thirty-minute orgasm. If I weren't having such a great time myself, I would definitely be jealous. Carolyn's ability to have repeated orgasms from this method of making love has improved over time.

In our first position, I am on top in the standard missionary position or on my side facing her. I support most of my weight, but rub my body against her, my chest lightly across her breasts, my pubic hair against hers to stimulate her clitoris. I kiss her and I begin to suck on her nipples. I suck each nipple as lightly as possible, running the tip of my tongue back and forth across the tip of the nipple, while counting in my head to 25 before switching from one to the other. I kiss her. I suck on her nipples. I rub my body against her. I repeat this cycle for five to seven minutes.

Next, we switch to the classic 69 position,

with her on top. She lays her head down close to my penis, looking at it, smelling it, but not touching it because that would get me excited to soon. She maneuvers her bottom so that I can put my tongue on her clitoris. I love to look at her and smell her. Her natural pheromones excite and stimulate me. She has a lot of pubic hair. She used to trim it, but I told her that I find it extremely stimulating to look at, so she stopped. I separate her pubic hair, moving it to the side with my fingers, exposing her clitoris and sliding the skin back to expose the most sensitive part, which I call the nub.

The clitoris has a hood that mostly covers it. Sometimes I'll stimulate it with the hood pulled back, but usually this is not a good idea because it is so sensitive. From this position the best approach is to lay the tip of my tongue flat against the side of the hood and move in wide circles across the top of the hood, around and across the front of the clitoris. I start with the lightest pressure that I can still feel with my tongue and gradually slightly increase it. Steady, repetitive motion (the same movement over and over), seems to work the best. Of course, this action can be done with your finger also.

I put my hands over her back and grab her bottom cheeks with both hands, spreading her cheeks so that I can see inside of her vagina and just enjoy the act of squeezing them. As I continue to work my tongue on her clitoris, I rub her shoulders and her back, massaging her muscles. Next, I have her raise the front part of her body up, so that her breasts are free. I cup them in my hands, squeezing them gently, lightly touching the sides. I roll her nipples between my thumb and middle finger, and lightly rub the top of the nipples with my index finger. While I'm touching her breasts, I continue to touch her clitoris with my tongue, using more pressure and a flatter surface moving in a circular motion. I use my tongue to push back the top of the hood and apply pressure to the nub underneath the hood. Then I switch back to a light circular motion on the front. After about eight minutes of this, we're ready for the next step.

Another good position is for her to lie on the bed with her legs spread apart, while I kneel on the floor on a pillow, off the side of the bed. I use my tongue to stimulate her clitoris and I also insert a finger in her vagina and press it down to rub against the muscles along the bottom of her vagina or put gentle pressure along the muscles on the sides. Sometimes I hold her breasts in my hand; sometimes I gently stroke her nipples while I'm stimulating her clitoris. The most difficult part about using this position is that I get tired quickly, and even a couple minutes seems like a long time to me, but is short for her. Another disadvantage is that my blood flows down into my big leg muscles. I want that blood to be available to pump up my penis. However, since this is a terrific position for Carolyn, we often start here. I try to make it about five minutes, then we switch to the classical 69 position where she's on top and I am laying on my back. It's important not to shortchange a woman here. Women take longer than men do to become fully aroused.

Next, Carolyn turns over on her back, leaning on several pillows. I lay next to her on her left. I kiss her. With my two hands I roll her nipples between my thumbs and index fingers, using my forefinger to rub the top of each nipple. Sometimes we hug from head to toe, kissing as we embrace. I press my leg between hers and up against her clitoris, as we lay on our sides. I do this for a few minutes, and then I move my head down and take the nipple of her left breast in my mouth and start to gently suck it, running my tongue over the tip while I suck. With my right hand, I roll her right nipple between my fingers. I move my left hand down to her vagina, inserting my index finger inside her. The back of my index finger presses against the bottom of her vagina at the surface of the entrance. My index finger extends deeper inside of her and leverages against her cervix. While I'm doing this, Carolyn touches her clitoris and rolls it under her finger or strokes it with light to medium pressure. She touches her own clitoris because it leaves me free to stimulate her nipples and vaginal muscles. She also knows what feels best on her clitoris, which requires a delicate touch.

One of the best effects of using these techniques is that Carolyn squeezes my index finger with her vaginal muscles. As she approaches orgasm, she squeezes harder, and I start to apply downward (varied with sideways) pressure with my index finger against her vaginal muscles. Over the past year and a half, the effect of all of this muscle building activity has been to develop stronger vaginal muscles. My penis is considerably thicker than my index finger. You can imagine how great it feels when those muscles squeeze it!

All of this motion with my finger in her vagina, my mouth on one nipple, and my fingers on the other nipple, starts lightly and gradually builds up, going on for five to fifteen minutes — building in momentum. It's important for me to start light with the nipples because that helps to maintain sensitivity, but also because my lips and my fingers will get too tired if I don't. As the intensity gradually builds, the muscles of her vagina gradually grip my finger harder and harder. I try to time things just so that I make an all out effort on her nipples at just the right time. This means sucking on the left breast and pulling and rolling the right breast with more intensity. Then her orgasm comes. Wow! It affects her whole body with rippling, pulsing shock waves. She turns toward me. I let go of her nipples and pull my fingers out of her vagina. I slide my left thigh up between her legs, with gentle pressure against her clitoris, and for a few moments, kiss and hold her, as her orgasm continues.

Then it's my turn

I like to look at her the most. I'm visual. I like her hand to play with my penis, lightly caressing my balls and pumping up and down on the shaft after it starts to get hard. I like to have my balls licked and very gently sucked. I like to have the tip of my penis sucked on and have her tongue rub on the triangle at the base of the tip.

I lie next to her while she plays with my penis. I look at her pubic hair. I turn and kiss her while I feel her inner thighs with my left hand. I lightly stroke her pubic hair as I stick my tongue in her mouth. She has another orgasm. I fantasize about when I was in high school and I wanted to feel-up teenage girls, wondering how their bushes felt.

When I start to get hard, I grab my penis just below the tip and pump on it vigorously. Next, I put some KY jelly on the tip of my penis. She climbs on top of me, and inserts my penis in her vagina. I just lay back and enjoy. She kisses me. She puts her tongue in my mouth. She rubs her nipples across the hair on my chest. She goes up and down, and around in circles. I put the flat palms of my hands on her breasts, squeeze her breasts and lightly squeeze her nipples between my fingers. I place my hands on her hips and push down to rub her clitoris harder against my pubic hair as she moves her pelvis forward towards my head and then backward. She has more orgasms. This goes on for five to ten minutes. I usually stay good and hard here because I'm relaxed on my back, and because of the squeezing motion of her vagina against the base of my penis.

Next, she climbs off, and I get on top in the standard missionary position. I always dry my penis off at this point, usually with an undershirt, so I can use my hand to pump it up. I look at her some more. I look at the pink lips, and the hair, which she does not trim or shave, and which is thick and luxurious. I imagine how it's going to feel to put my penis inside of her. I stroke my penis more. It gets stiffer. With my left hand, I run my fingers up and down her inner thighs, especially at the point where her crotch meets her leg. I lightly touch her clitoris. I slowly slide my finger into her vagina. Once inside I curve it downward and apply gentle pressure to the band of muscles that run along the bottom of her vagina, then I curve to the right and to the left, gently stroking those muscles. Then I extend my finger full length, turn it over and curve it upward to hit her cervix and the top of the vagina.

All of this is very exciting for me. I wet the tip with KY jelly, and Carolyn guides it inside her. I put it in as far as it will go and try to rub my pubic hair against her clitoris. She squeezes with her pelvic muscles. I like to hold myself up off of her when we first start out so that I can watch my penis going in and out.

After a few minutes I get tired and pull out. I dry off my penis again and repeat the previous steps of looking at her and pumping it up again. Slightly rested, I wet the tip again with KY jelly and reinsert. This goes on for a few times, until I build up to a climax. The rest stops are good for both of us. Her pelvic muscles get rested, and I build up my strength and get my wind back.

As I approach orgasm, how I feel depends on how horny I am and how much time has passed since we last had sex. At my best, with my penis very hard, I feel powerful. I'm on top.

Carolyn is under me moaning and shivering with repeated orgasms. She has a steady, slippery, tight grip on my penis. I feel her whole body against mine. After my orgasm, sometimes I roll off of her and lay exhausted by her side (sometimes I just lay still and close on top of her for a few minutes). I feel the endorphins released flow from the center of my body out throughout my entire body. It's wonderful!

I feel close and connected when we have sex. Sex is bonding for us. I always feel safe and accepted with her. The first time we had sex, I worried about how I would perform — whether my penis would get hard or not. I had some trouble the first time, but the emotional safety and acceptance that I felt with Carolyn allowed me to quickly overcome that the next time we made love.

When we have sex early in the morning, right after I wake up, sometimes I don't have an orgasm, and sometimes I do. It depends on how satisfied I feel, how relaxed I am, and how well I've slept. What I like about morning sex is that I always have a great hard-on, which I want to put inside of Carolyn. I like the feeling of being close to each other. Sometimes I'll spoon up to her from behind as she lies on her side facing away from me, and slip my penis inside her from behind, but she usually climbs on top after I've lubricated the tip of my penis with KY jelly.

She said

I'd like to comment both as a woman and as a therapist.

Making love with Wes has been like a dream come true for me. I love the way Wes and I make love. I have a strong sex drive; I've been interested in sexual expression since puberty. It's an important aspect of my relationship. I've also craved the safety and validation of intimacy all of my life. I didn't know what it was I wanted exactly, but this is reasonably descriptive, and comes close to naming what I was looking for.

Making love with Wes is so good for me because it's physically and emotionally satisfying. It's physically satisfying because he knows exactly what I like and need to have an orgasm. He not only wants to pleasure me, but also feels good about providing so much pleasure to me. It's part of his own excitement and arousal to do this for me. He also takes pride in performing well and so he takes good care of himself. Thankfully, he isn't bogged down in simultaneous orgasms or such extremes of so-called perfect sex that he becomes lost in the performance rather than the expression of love and nurturing. Making love with Wes is emotionally satisfying because it's an expression of closeness, warmth, love, and nurturing. He's also accepting of me; he likes me as I am, which fuels me to be my true self. I feel deep satisfaction in having this.

I want to make a few comments about the sex itself. Making sex a priority in our relationship is not something we force, but it is something we protect. We both have a strong interest in sexual expression, so its prominence is natural for us. I usually need a transitional period as we shift into focusing on each other sexually. Again, we match so well in our daily rhythm it's easy for us to follow our instincts and desires, knowing the other is pretty closely attuned.

We both like me to have an orgasm first. Wes likes it because he has a chance to relax longer, and because my orgasm helps my muscles contract, which adds to his physical pleasure. I like it because it allows me to have multiple orgasms. I'm not able to have an orgasm from intercourse easily. I have only twice in my life – purely by accident. Usually I need more direct stimulation on my clitoris than intercourse provides. However, once I've had an orgasm, I'm sensitive to any stimulation, and intercourse easily triggers multiple orgasms. This adds to my satisfaction tremendously!

While we're not against changing what we do, it feels good to know that we have a range of activities that we know works. The repetition of the activities is not monotonous to me; the safety and predictability actually add to my satisfaction.

Part of my satisfaction definitely relates to satisfying Wes. It's deeply satisfying to give him pleasure and help him take care of his sexual needs. The mutuality of our relationship adds further emotional safety to the climate of our relationship.

Now a few comments as a therapist. Even though we're both reasonably balanced in so-called male/female characteristics within ourselves individually, like many men and women, Wes is more focused on the physical "ness" of things; I'm prone to focus on the mental/emotional aspects of life. When he told you about sexual potency, he spoke of the physical part of potency. So I want to say a word about mental/emotional aspects of sexual potency. It's essential that you feel good about yourself, feel validated by your partner, and be fit. He needed to work on both aspects for his natural potency to return. It didn't take long either! The two aspects fuel each other. Taking care of yourself physically helps you feel better about yourself, and feeling good about yourself leads you to do good things for yourself. It's impossible to separate the two. In some instances impotency is purely physical, caused by diabetes, cardiovascular disease, or heavy use of alcohol. And certain medication and drugs can cause impotency. But, many times emotional turmoil causes sexual impotency. You must be in an emotionally safe environment where you feel valued and appreciated to realize your sexual potential. Having a poor or mediocre relationship doesn't provide this kind of emotional safety. Having a great relationship is the only climate that can provide this kind of safety.

I also want to point out the wonderful example Wes gave about his earliest sexually stimulating experiences. He's visual, as are many people, particularly men, and when he spied on his friend's sister in the eighth grade, he most likely became highly aroused by the sight. The vision of her pubic hair is forever fixed in his mind as arousing to him. There's nothing perverse about this. Things like this that become fixed in your arousal pattern are innocent, normal, and natural. Arousal patterns like – in Wes's case – seeing bushy dark public hair is not an indication of less interest in your partner, or less desire for mutual, sexually satisfying activity. They're rarely harmful to anyone, and the partner would do well to work these types of arousal into their behavior. Of course, sometimes people can be dreadfully harmed in his or her childhood around issues that are sexual, and the extreme of this situation could result in danger. It's a matter of degree. If you've gotten your head straight, you'll never stay in any relationship where you sense a dangerous perversion. I would also add that Wes's father must have handled this sensitive situation with understanding, because it didn't turn into a terrible memory for him.

I'm not saying that spying in the window at anyone is okay. It's an intrusive act, and that's wrong. But a young person who's overwhelmed with sexual curiosity isn't born knowing that. And they're not born knowing how to cope with such overwhelming desires. When things like this happen, you must correct the behavior, explaining that it's not acceptable, without damaging the self-esteem of the young person. Their embarrassment at being caught, along with the information that you give them about it being wrong, is enough to change the behavior. The fact that you care enough to guide a young person's behavior in a loving and respectful way will change their behavior. It's also important to supply an acceptable outlet to satisfy their sexual curiosity. If you don't, they'll find a way to satisfy it, and it may not be the best way.

The converse of this kind of situation can happen also. It's more common for females to become frightened somehow by their first sexual stimulation. If something does happen during childhood that frightens the person, the behavior fixed could remain tension-filled, even though, in the context of a good relationship, the behavior would cause no harm. To avoid depriving you or your partner of satisfying experiences respect your individual differences.

The information above is offered in the hope that those of you confused about satisfying a partner can resolve your confusion. Both of us lacked adequate sexual information earlier in our lives. We struggled to have satisfying sexual relationships. Please afford yourself a continuing sexual education so that you, too, can have great sex in the context of a great marriage.

10

Special Boundaries: Rituals, Ceremonies, and Symbols

Getting Your Marriage Off to a Great Start

Great marriages deserve great beginnings. If you feel certain that you've found your perfect partner, it's time to plan what to do next.

The First Task of Every Marriage

Judith Wallerstein, author of The Good Marriage (Houghton Mifflin, 1995), has been doing research on the effects of divorce on children for 25 years. Having determined that divorce wreaks havoc on the lives of children, Wallerstein decided that we have to get a better grip on having successful marriages. Recently she conducted research on 50 self-described, good marriages. In doing her research, she defined nine tasks that every marriage must master in order to have a good marriage. We want to tell you about the first task.

The first of those nine tasks is that the individuals in a new marriage – beginning when the relationship takes a turn toward marriage – must shift their primary loyalty from their family of origin to their partner and unit together as a couple and later a family. In order to do so you must have good couple boundaries. To have good couple boundaries you must begin by having good individual boundaries.

Personal Boundaries

Boundaries are the limits you will tolerate for your own and others' behavior. Everything we talked to you about – having a strong sense of self, knowing how you think and feel, thinking for yourself, matching your behavior to your beliefs and values, acting with intention, liking yourself, and the behavior you'll accept from others – are the boundaries that define you. We've asked you to define who you are so you can be clear about your boundaries. The most successful people have strong boundaries that neither allow unacceptable intrusiveness by others, nor isolation from others. People with strong and clear boundaries neither have to borrow a self from others nor feel a need to foist their identity on others. People with clear boundaries don't confuse others about what their boundaries are.

The most basic, fundamental element of great marriages is individuals with clear and strong boundaries. When two people with clear and strong boundaries match on those boundaries – the 16 differences that make a difference are types of boundaries – and they have strong boundaries about the other four crucial questions, they have the ability to have good couple boundaries. It takes good couple boundaries to master the first task of marriage.

Couple Boundaries

When you become a couple and turn your intention toward marriage the world must be informed of the birth of your new status and intention to commit to one another. This is another circumstance where you have to back up your words with action.

Because of boundary issues and legal issues, we believe that marriage is important. Living with someone never has the same level of commitment and the benefits of a great marriage cannot happen without commitment and emotional safety. Living with someone cannot give you the same level of synergy that marriage gives you. We believe that marriage is a boundary – it's a special boundary that we'll talk more about in a moment.

The task of shifting your primary loyalty to you and your partner as a couple and the beginning of a new family requires setting boundaries from the point that you decide you'll marry. When you can be clear about this first boundary as a couple many other things about starting your lives together will clarify.

When we got married four years ago we had to set boundaries as a couple. It didn't matter that we'd been married before. We had to master the first marital task, as does everyone who wants a great marriage.

First, we encountered family members that wanted to tell us how to have our wedding. Then we had other family members that wanted us to honeymoon at their house with them. Then we had family that wanted us to take annual vacations with the rest of the family – every year. Other issues came up around how and where to live, how to act, how to parent, where to sit at ballgames. And on and on. It's pretty amazing how others want you to do and act as they believe proper and think it strange that you may have your own way – or never even consider that you may have your own ideas about what you intend to do.

When we first got together, Wes had never really heard the term boundaries used the way we're describing boundaries. In fact, boundaries – or a lack of them – are a big issue in his family of origin. But Wes is a quick study and he caught on fast. And he felt much better for it, too. In no time we were acting in our own best interest as a couple. It felt great.

Carolyn had already had plenty of practice both in her own life and as a therapist in setting limits and helping others to set limits.

Setting couple boundaries takes a unified couple. You will fail your partner if you fail to shift your primary loyalty to your partner and the two of you as a couple.

We handled each of these incidences with consistency and firm determination and eventually the fury died down. It flares up now and again, and we find ourselves taking a deep breath and setting limits again.

Setting limits and having clear boundaries empowers us to live our lives exactly the way we want to live our lives. We have control of our own lives. People that don't have control of their own lives are depressed, angry, and resentful. It doesn't occur to them that it's up to them to take control and set limits. Realizing that it's up to them is liberating and empowering.

We just said over and over that we would handle our own wedding plans. Something about weddings brings out the craziness in every family. Everyone thinks they know best. Many family members feel the wedding belongs to them. As with advice about anything, we'd listen to others' opinions and then decide for ourselves what we intended to do. That was no small task at times. Have you ever seen grown adults manipulating, and insinuating, and contorting to get their way? The guilt trips can be amazing. Well they tried everything. But no one can control you unless you let them. We just held a steady course and had the wedding we wanted to have.

Have the wedding you want to have. It's your wedding. Start your marriage off right and set limits.

As for the honeymoon – we would never consider having our honeymoon with others. And they thought we were off our rockers. After all, we'd each been married before – what's the big deal? Well it is a big deal. We wanted to be alone. We wanted to follow our own schedule. We wanted to go somewhere different.

Have the honeymoon you want to have. It's your honeymoon. Begin your marriage right – set its tone.

The annual family vacation was a big issue. It took months to convince others we meant business and would take our vacations when and how and where we wanted. Of course others took it personally. They didn't consider that Carolyn spends her work time with unhappy couples and families and spending her vacation that way wouldn't be any vacation for her. They didn't consider that we wanted to go different places and see new things. They didn't consider that we have so much fun together that we don't need a huge crowd or that we might want to spend quality fun time with each other. They didn't consider that we wanted to do something different than they wanted to do. So we just stayed the course and finally the roar died down. The family has discovered that our having our vacation how and where and when we wanted didn't mean we didn't love them. It didn't mean that we never wanted to see them. They realize that we mean business and that we've managed to see them, at times, too.

Carolyn can remember how horrible starting her first marriage was when the relatives
kept fighting about where they would stay during visits and how much they'd see of each family. She vowed that she'd never put that kind of
pressure on her children and their families.
Keeping that promise to herself in mind,
Christmas at her house comes in the afternoon
after the young families have had some private
time together or after Christmas Eve and morning with their wives' families. It's begun a new
tradition. By the time everyone gets to her
house all the other families feel satisfied and no
one has to hurry. It's worked out beautifully.
And when our married children are in town for
Christmas we share them with each other (the
parents) and have us to each other's houses.
Our tradition setting is a boundary.

Other common day-to-day boundaries
include asking people to call before they drop
by, answering the phone when you want rather
than whenever it rings, or being able to excuse
yourself from a phone call when you're finished
talking. Asking people to call during certain
times when a new baby comes home and only to
come over when pre-arranged is a boundary. Of
course, you'll want to extend the same courte-
sies to others. Honor your own and others'
boundaries.

New couples and new families must forge
and protect their own boundaries and traditions. Start at the very beginning to set limits
and have clear boundaries.

Back your partner up – even if your mother is pulling every trick in the book to get her way. We all loved our mothers first, but you must shift your primary loyalty to your new family. Remind your mother of how much she would have wanted that for herself. Gentle and friendly firmness will help others respect the boundaries that you set for yourselves. Your partner, your couplehood, your new family come first.

Special Boundaries – Rituals, Ceremonies, and Symbols

It is ironic to us that, today, as we write to you about special boundaries, the world is watching the funeral of Princess Diana. Funerals serve a purpose. Their ritual and ceremony offer us an opportunity to make a transition in our lives.

Funerals are an example of special boundaries. It was a funeral that heightened Carolyn's awareness years ago of the importance of rituals, ceremonies, and symbols – all special boundaries. Carolyn believed, before the funeral of her young mother-in-law, the grandmother of her children, that funerals seemed a waste. It was in living through the grief of her mother-in-law's sudden death that Carolyn learned how important it is to say good-bye – how important it is to take a moment and have closure.

It is through rituals, ceremonies, and symbols that we communicate to each other the changes in our status in life. We celebrate a baby's birth with birthdays. We reaffirm our spiritual beliefs through christenings. We recognize growth, gaining maturity, and independence through graduations and certain religious ceremonies. We say good-bye at wakes and funerals and offer one another emotional support for our grief and loss.

And we celebrate the significant change in status of individuals when they vow to live together in marriage with weddings and receptions. It is at a wedding that a couple says to others that they have committed to each other and future children to live together as husband and wife. After the wedding, it is wedding rings that symbolize those vows. Rings help us communicate our wedded status to others, serving to lessen the complexities of relationships.

It is at our wedding that we demonstrate to others and help them recognize the change in our status to a new family unit. Weddings afford us an opportunity to set a new boundary. Rings assist in setting that boundary. Honeymoons, alone, set a boundary of privacy for the beginning of this new primary unit – a new family.

We believe in weddings and marriage. Great marriages start with the right partners, engagements, and weddings.

He said

We decided to have our wedding on February 12, 1994, about five months after we met. The father-in-law of Carolyn's son, who, along with his wife, is a friend of ours too, conducted the religious ceremony. We had our wedding and reception at Paul's on the South River (a wonderful restaurant in Annapolis). The food and drink were outstanding; smoked salmon and chocolate covered strawberries were two of my favorite choices. We had lots of flowers. The wedding cake came in two pieces with white rolled Austrian frosting draped over each piece. The inside was a yellow cake with raspberry filling. David and Ginger Hildebrand played music – light classical, traditional wedding, old colonial, and Chesapeake Bay water music. About 75 people attended – relatives from California and Colorado, our five children, and our friends. Carolyn wore a tea length, tailored white dress, and I wore a dark blue suit. One of the best things we did at our wedding was to hand around several disposable cameras with flashes. Because everyone had a slightly different view of the wedding and the people there, we got some fantastic pictures. Our picture album is full of super pictures.

One of the issues we had to discuss and work out before the wedding was about rings. I had never worn any type of ring, and at first didn't want one. Carolyn convinced me that a wedding ring is an extraordinarily important and meaningful symbol. Wearing a ring is an outward sign in our society that you're married. It sets boundaries in your relationships with other people – in my case, other women. I can remember that toward the end of my previous marriage, my ex-wife took off her ring. Strangely, I noticed it in one of the kitchen cabinets. At the time, I tried not to think too much about what that meant, but now I can see clearly that, of course, she meant our marriage was over. Similarly, Carolyn's first husband managed to lose his wedding ring about two months after their wedding. She thinks he did it because he was only 19 and wasn't finished fooling around.

We had some serious problems with the weather the entire week of our wedding. The Baltimore airport froze over and was shut down just as the plane carrying Carolyn's mother was due to land. She was diverted to North Carolina for two days. The roads iced up so badly the night of the wedding that, when we drove to the airport the next day along I-97, we passed dozens of cars abandoned along side the road. What a great time to head for Florida for a week on our honeymoon!

I can remember feeling good, not nervous, throughout the whole wedding ceremony. Carolyn had done a wonderful job organizing everything. The people from Paul's were exceptionally capable. They practically ran the wedding for us. I was surprised at how many people attended, sitting around tables, when I walked out on the small platform where the ceremony was performed. Carolyn's three sons and my son and daughter stood up for us as witnesses.

Even though we weren't in church, the ceremony was a fairly standard religious ceremony. We promised to love and honor each other. Between ourselves, we promised to learn how to negotiate our conflicts.

There were two moments when we were up on the platform that I thought were wonderful. As we cut the wedding cake, we fed each other and then kissed. This was delicious. When we were posing for pictures, someone said, "Kiss the bride again!" I gave Carolyn a bent over kiss like a sailor back from World War II. When we saw the pictures of this kiss, both of our mothers were in the photo with a "Wow! What are they doing in public?" look. It was wonderful.

We socialized with our guests. We stayed together as we went around the room. In fact, we stayed together throughout the whole ceremony and reception. I noticed at another wedding that the couple split up during the reception. I remember from my first wedding that my ex-wife and I split up at the reception. It's a small, but telling sign.

Weddings can be fairly stressful. So many relatives! Our kids came through for us big time with a wonderful wedding present. On our wedding night, we planned to stay at our house and leave for Florida early the next morning. When we were planning the wedding, with so many things to consider, we forgot one extremely important point: both of our mothers would be sleeping in the house with us — one in the next bedroom! On our wedding night! After the wedding, we went back to our house and got together in the living room with friends and family to open wedding gifts. We opened a gift from our kids – a card with some writing on it that promised a night in the presidential suite at a waterfront hotel in Annapolis, a window looking across the icy water toward the Naval Academy with all of the moored boats, room service, and an enormous bathroom and tub. I can remember reading this card and, for the first few minutes, not realizing what it meant. I think Carolyn must have had a rather puzzled look on her face too, because one of the kids leaned over, pointed at the card, and said, "It's for tonight!" The realization that we could escape from everyone sunk in. We wouldn't have to take our mothers to the airport first thing in the morning. We could just think about ourselves and be together. We were packed, out of the house, and on our way to Annapolis in about 45 minutes.

She said

I loved our wedding. Even though we had some tense moments the day and evening before (weddings bring out every family's craziness), we were able to have our wedding exactly the way we wanted it. Everything about the wedding and reception was exactly as I'd planned. We were deeply happy and very much in love. What can be better than being with your perfect partner, being happy and in love, and with your friends and family celebrating with wonderful food, in a beautiful place, hearing beautiful music? What a beginning.

Our honeymoon continued to be exactly as we wanted. As Wes said, we got to start it sooner than we planned, which was the best thing that could have happened to us. We were both being so practical we had overlooked getting off by ourselves on our wedding night. The kids didn't overlook it though; they came through for us.

We went to the airport the next morning for a flight to Orlando. The weather we left was dreadful, as Wes said. (I picked our wedding date because it was Valentine's Day and because I'm usually miserable by February. The winter starts to get me down by then, and I dream of spring. With our anniversary in February, we now have a reason to do something fantastic every year, which I thought would improve the month immensely.) We arrived in Orlando after a short flight. The weather was magnificent — 75 and sunny.

Our honeymoon was a package we got through American Express Travel Service. It included everything – the flight, ground transportation, the hotel, and unlimited passes to all of the Disney theme parks for the eight days we were there. It was a convenient and economical way to arrange the trip. I'm into making life as easy and wonderful as it can be, and we planned this trip — as we did our wedding — to be just what we wanted. And we weren't disappointed. The trip was the best we'd ever had.

We spent eight days going to all of the Disney theme parks. (I learned that Disney World in Orlando has more honeymoons than any other place in the world.) We'd usually get up early in the morning and head for whichever theme park was open early to vacationers staying at the Disney hotels. We had a tour book we'd bought in preparation for the trip — Fodor's Walt Disney World for Adults, by Rita Aero. The tour book gives you some great ideas about what and how to see things in each of the parks. We'd spend the morning, lunch, and early afternoon at Magic Kingdom, MGM Studios, or Epcot, and then we'd go back to the hotel. Mid and late afternoons we usually made love, took a nap, and then either went swimming or to the Jacuzzi. At night we'd return to a theme park for dinner and night shows. We had a ball!

Without a doubt, where we stayed was as magical as the theme parks. Disney's Grand Floridian Hotel is spectacular. It was so beautiful that sometimes we just stayed there.

Our wedding and honeymoon were exactly the way to start our marriage out right.

WARNING

Watch out! Your friends and family may be extremely jealous when your life works out so wonderfully for you! (Of course, they may also want the best for you. People do have mixed feelings at times.) When people feel jealous they can act in many different ways, including trying to get you back in line again!

She said

More than one person has actually ridiculed me for having love and marriage all figured out. Fortunately, I had the presence of mind to say I wasn't going to apologize for having gotten things figured out for myself. I don't feel one bit guilty! I feel wonderful. I'm having a wonderful time, and I feel deeply grateful!

It's interesting that one of my sons found this to be true also. When I told him that this business about working at making your relationship work was a lie, he said he thought so too. He said that people say to his wife and him that they can't be real. They get along so well, are best friends, don't fight, and are so happy that people don't believe it can be so. Rather than ask themselves what must be wrong in their relationships, they deny that it's possible to have such a great relationship. Friends of mine actually said to me once that they (my son and his wife) must be phony to be so happy.

Be careful. If you're tempted to resist the idea of having all of this happiness, think about why. We want to give hope to you. We're not gloating! With all humility, this is what's possible. This is what you can have. Believe us. If we can work through the issues we had and get where we've gotten, so can you!

Choosing the right marriage partner is the most important decision you'll make in your life. A successful marriage is the foundation for all of the other successes in your life.

We hope the information we've given you in this book will have provided you meaningful guidance in your search for your perfect partner and a great marriage. It has been our desire to give you the beginning of new hope and confidence toward finding your perfect partner and a great marriage.

If you'd like structured guidance to make your way through this process, we've written three workbooks designed to give you that. Perfect Partners™: Find Your Perfect Partner Step-By-Step is for singles looking for their perfect partner. Perfect Partners™: When You Think You've Found Your Perfect Partner Step-By-Step is for singles that believe they've found their perfect partner. Perfect Partners™: Should You Stay or Should You Leave? Step-By-Step is for married couples in troubled marriages that want help to make this very difficult decision.

For those of you searching for your perfect partner and a great marriage we say congratulations. Please accept our very best wishes for a lifetime of happiness. Welcome to an ever-growing group of individuals and couples unwilling to accept anything less than the best.

Suggested Reading

Branden, Nathaniel. <u>The Six Pillars of Self-Esteem</u>, New York, NY: Bantam Books, 1995.

Covey, Stephen R. <u>The 7 Habits of Highly Effective People</u>: Powerful Lessons in Personal Change, New York, NY: Simon & Schuster Inc., 1989.

Delaney, Gayle. <u>Living Your Dreams</u> (rev. ed.), San Francisco, CA: Harper & Row, 1988.

Dyer, Dr. Wayne W. <u>Your Sacred Self: Making the Decision to Be Free</u>, New York, NY: Harper Collins Publishers, Inc., 1995.

Jackson, Carole. <u>Color Me Beautiful</u>, New York, NY: Ballantine Books, 1984.

Jackson, Carole. <u>Color for Men</u>, New York, NY: Ballantine Books, 1987.

Puhn, Adele. <u>The 5 Day Miracle Diet</u>, New York, NY: Random House, Inc., 1996.

The Authors

Carolyn and Wes met after 25 years of surviving typical hit-or-miss relationships. After a variety of miseries (much time and energy, marriages to the wrong partner, hard work to make those marriages work, undermined self-confidence, unhappy children), they found a pragmatic approach that helped them sift out the wrong prospects and find each other. Their hope that marriage didn't have to be hard work with the wrong partner allowed them to question the norm. They fell in love joyfully, romantically, and effortlessly, without any emotional roller-coaster rides.

As a therapist, Carolyn has helped hundreds of individuals, couples, and families surmount their relationship problems. In guiding many through the processes they used to find each other she has helped them to discover their Perfect Partners™.

Carolyn is an Advanced Practice Nurse who is licensed to practice as a Nurse Psychotherapist. She received her BS in Nursing from Johns Hopkins University in 1979 and her MS in Psychiatric Nursing from the

University of Maryland at Baltimore in 1988. She is certified by the American Nurses' Association as a Specialist in Psychiatric Nursing.

Having worked in in-patient psychiatric services in several hospitals, with both the private and public sectors of inner cities and the suburbs, Carolyn has more recently done emergency psychiatric evaluations for her community hospital making referrals and doing crisis intervention. As the hospital's psychiatric representative, she has been interviewed on numerous occasions for newspaper articles on mental health and for a local news/commentary TV show on community mental health issues. She has also been the hospital's representative on many state and local mental health task-force committees. She has been in private practice since 1988.

Wes received his BS in Physics and Math from the University of Illinois in 1970. He received his MS in Physics from the University of Illinois in 1972. He has a teaching certificate from the University of Oregon, and in 1986 he completed his MBA at the University of Maryland. He's been a teacher, an engineer, a computer programmer and a manager, and specializes in database software development.

Carolyn is the mother of three happily married grown sons and married for the third time. Wes is the father of a son and daughter and this is his second marriage. Carolyn and Wes have been happily married for four years.

𝔓erfect 𝔓artnersTM/SM

Books, Workbooks & Consultation

Order next page and send to or call:

BookMasters, Inc.
P.O. Box 388
Ashland, OH 44805
Book Order Telephone: 800/247-6553
Email Order: order@bookmasters.com
http://www.bookmasters.com

Visit Carolyn & Wes Huff at their
website
http://www.perfectpartners.net

For Ordering Book & Workbooks
Please Send:

The Book – Perfect Partners™ Make Your
Hopes and Dreams for a Great Marriage
Come True (The full text from which the
workbooks were derived, including our
our personal example of great sex). $24.95
(Available 1st quarter of 1998)　　　　_____

The Workbook – Perfect Partners™: Find
Your Perfect Partner Step-By-Step (For
singles that are looking for their perfect
partner) $18.95　　　　_____

The Workbook – Perfect Partners™: When
You Think You've Found Your Perfect Partner
Step-By-Step (For singles that want to know
if they have found their perfect partner; the
sequel to the previous workbook) $18.95
*This workbook is $10.00 when you buy it
together with Find Your Perfect Partner
Step-By-Step　　　　_____

The Workbook – Perfect Partners™: Should
You Stay or Should You Leave? Step-By-Step
(For married couples in a troubled marriage)
$18.95　　　　_____

State Tax Ohio Residents add 6%　　　　_____

Shipping & Handling	
$0 – 30.00	$5.95
30.01 – 60.00	7.95
60.01 – 90.00	9.95
90.01 – 150.00	12.95
150.01 – 250.00	15.95
250.00 +	Please call

TOTAL　　　　_____

-continued next page-

Please enclose check or money order
for total - or

_____

Please charge total to my credit card
(VISA or MC)

_____

Account # _____ Exp. Date _____

Signature _____

To: Name_____
     Address_____
     City, State, Zip_____

_____

Phone & best time to call_____

_____

*Please see next page for ordering
phone consultation.

To Order Phone Consultation

Please use this form by mail to:
Perfect PartnersTM/SM
EMPOWERMENT SOLUTIONS INC.
550 M Ritchie Highway
Suite 142
Severna Park, MD 21146

or call (410) 647-6745 and leave a message to arrange
one hour of phone consultation for help with per-
sonalizing the Perfect PartnersTM/SM process.
$250.00. We will return your call to arrange a
time convenient to your schedule.

You will receive a free Perfect PartnersTM/SM book or
workbook of your choice when ordering phone
consultation. We will mail your choice to you priority mail prior to our phone consultation.

Name: _____

Address: _____

_____

Phone: _____

Best time to call: _____

Name of free book choice: _____

If paying by check or money order, please
enclose with this order form.
If paying by credit card (MC, VISA), we will bill
you at the time your appointment is
arranged.